Regulatory Compliance in the Healthcare Industry: Navigating the Complexities

Dr. Akash Sharma

Ms. Vriti Gamta

Mr. Gaurav Luthra

Contents

List of Figures

List of Tables

Preface

elcome to **"Regulatory Compliance in the Healthcare Industry: Navigating the Complexities."** This book serves as a comprehensive guide for healthcare professionals, compliance officers, administrators, and anyone involved in the intricate world of regulatory compliance in healthcare.

In today's healthcare landscape, compliance with laws, regulations, and industry standards is paramount. The healthcare industry is subject to a complex web of regulatory requirements, ranging from patient privacy and safety to billing and coding practices, pharmaceutical regulations, research ethics, and more. Navigating these complexities can be challenging and requires a deep understanding of the ever-evolving regulatory landscape.

This book is designed to provide a holistic view of regulatory compliance in healthcare, covering a wide range of topics and addressing the unique challenges faced by healthcare organizations. It explores the roles of key regulatory bodies, such as the FDA, CMS, and HIPAA, and delves into the significance of compliance in promoting patient safety, data security, and quality of care.

Throughout the chapters, we delve into the essential components of a robust compliance program, including establishing policies and procedures, conducting risk assessments, and implementing effective internal controls. We explore the critical role of compliance officers and their responsibilities in ensuring adherence to regulations and promoting an ethical culture within organizations.

The book also explores the intricacies of healthcare privacy and security regulations, covering issues like patient confidentiality, data breach response, and the widespread use and security of electronic health records. It examines the compliance requirements specific to pharmaceuticals and medical devices, including drug approval processes, product safety, and labeling compliance.

In addition, the book plunges into the issues and implications of compliance in research and clinical trials, long-term care institutions, health insurance, and worldwide healthcare operations. It covers emerging trends, such as the impact of technology advancements and changing healthcare policies, and provides insights into building effective compliance programs, conducting audits, and responding to investigations.

Each chapter is packed with practical information, real-world case studies, and best practices, offering valuable guidance for healthcare professionals seeking to navigate the complex terrain of regulatory compliance. Additionally, tables, checklists, and resources are provided throughout the book to aid in understanding and implementing compliance initiatives.

It is our hope that this book will serve as a valuable resource and companion for healthcare professionals as they navigate the intricacies of regulatory compliance. By embracing compliance best practices and fostering a culture of integrity, healthcare organizations can enhance patient safety, protect sensitive information, mitigate risks, and ultimately improve the quality of care provided.

We encourage you to dive into the chapters, engage with the content, and adapt the strategies and recommendations to your unique healthcare setting. Together, let us embark on this journey to ensure regulatory compliance, promote ethical practices, and build a stronger, more compliant healthcare industry.

Happy reading!

About the Author

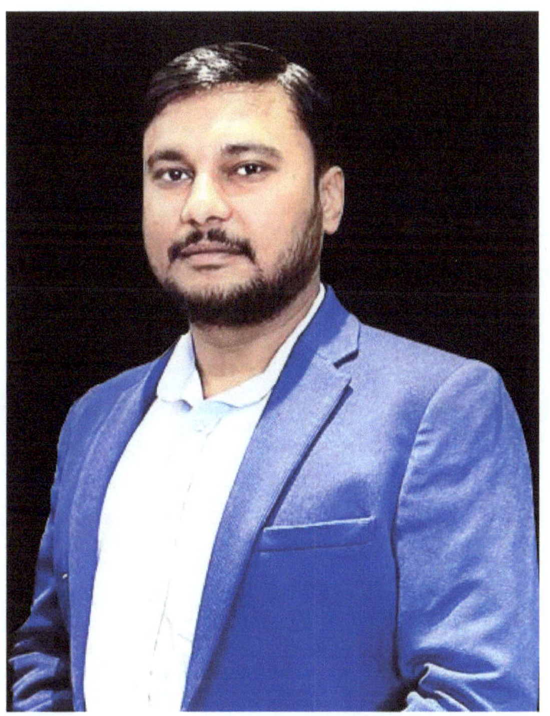

Dr. Akash Sharma is a highly accomplished professional in the field of Regulatory Affairs and Quality Management System for the medical device industry. With a strong academic background and extensive industry experience, Dr. Sharma brings a wealth of knowledge and expertise to the subject of Risk Management in this comprehensive guide. Dr. Sharma holds a Ph.D. & M.Tech in Mechanical Engineering. His research focus has been on the Application of Risk Management Principles in the Medical Device Industry, and he has published over 35 research papers in reputable journals and two books regarding Risk Management and Risk-Based Quality Management in the Healthcare Industry.

Additionally, he has actively participated in more than 15 international conferences, where he has shared his insights and contributed to the advancements in the field. With a career spanning over seven years, Dr. Sharma has gained valuable experience in regulatory affairs and quality management systems. He has a deep understanding of regulatory requirements, particularly in relation to the European Medical Device Regulation (EU MDR), CE certification and ISO 13485 for quality management systems. His expertise also extends to risk management, specifically in accordance with ISO 14971, the internationally recognized standard for managing risks associated with medical devices.

Currently serving as the Regulatory Affairs Manager and Management Representative at KAULMED PRIVATE LIMITED (KAUL-Medizintechnik GmbH), Dr. Sharma plays a vital role in ensuring compliance with regulatory standards and driving quality initiatives within the organization. His hands-on experience in navigating the complexities of regulatory requirements and implementing effective risk management practices makes him a trusted authority in the field.

Dr. Sharma's passion for the medical device industry and his commitment to patient safety and product quality are evident in his work. Through this book, he shares his knowledge, practical insights, and best practices to guide professionals in the medical device industry towards successful risk management practices.

Dr. Akash Sharma's expertise, research contributions, and extensive industry experience make him a valuable resource for professionals seeking to enhance their understanding of risk management in the medical device industry. His dedication to excellence and continuous learning make him a trusted authority in the field.

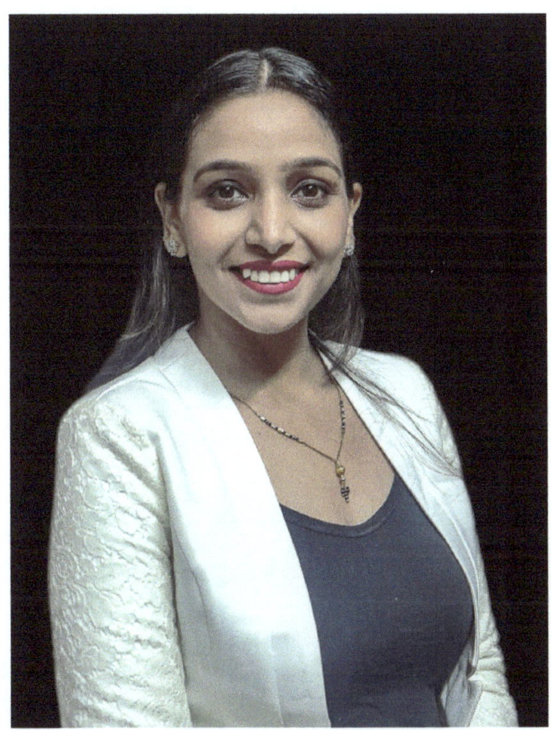

Vriti Gamta is a talented book author with a strong background in the healthcare industry. She holds a Master's degree in Pharmacy with a specialization in Drug Regulatory Affairs (DRA). With over four years of experience in Regulatory Affairs and Quality Management System, Vriti has established herself as an expert in navigating the complex regulatory landscape of the healthcare sector. Vriti's expertise lies in ensuring compliance with regulations and standards related to medical devices and pharmaceutical products. She is particularly knowledgeable in the European Union Medical Device Regulation (EU MDR), which sets out the requirements for placing medical devices on the market within the EU. In addition to her regulatory affairs proficiency, Vriti is well-versed in Quality Management Systems, specifically ISO 13485. This standard outlines the requirements for a comprehensive quality management system for the design, development, production, and distribution of medical devices.

Vriti has also developed a keen understanding of risk management principles, particularly ISO 14971. This international standard provides guidelines for identifying, evaluating, and controlling risks associated with medical devices throughout their lifecycle. Her commitment to advancing knowledge in her field is evident through her publications of two books guiding healthcare professionals about Risk Management in Healthcare Industry and Risk-Based Quality Management System, as well as seven papers in international journals. These publications showcase her ability to conduct research, analyze data, and contribute to the scientific community within the healthcare industry.

Currently, Vriti holds the position of Regulatory Affairs Executive at KAULMED PRIVATE LIMITED (KAUL-Medizintechnik GmbH), where she plays a crucial role in ensuring regulatory compliance and maintaining high-quality standards for the organization's medical devices and pharmaceutical products.

Vriti Gamta's combination of academic qualifications, extensive experience, and research contributions makes her a respected authority in Regulatory Affairs and Quality Management Systems within the healthcare industry. As a book author, she may reach a larger audience and impart her wisdom and insights, offering invaluable advice to both experts and enthusiasts.

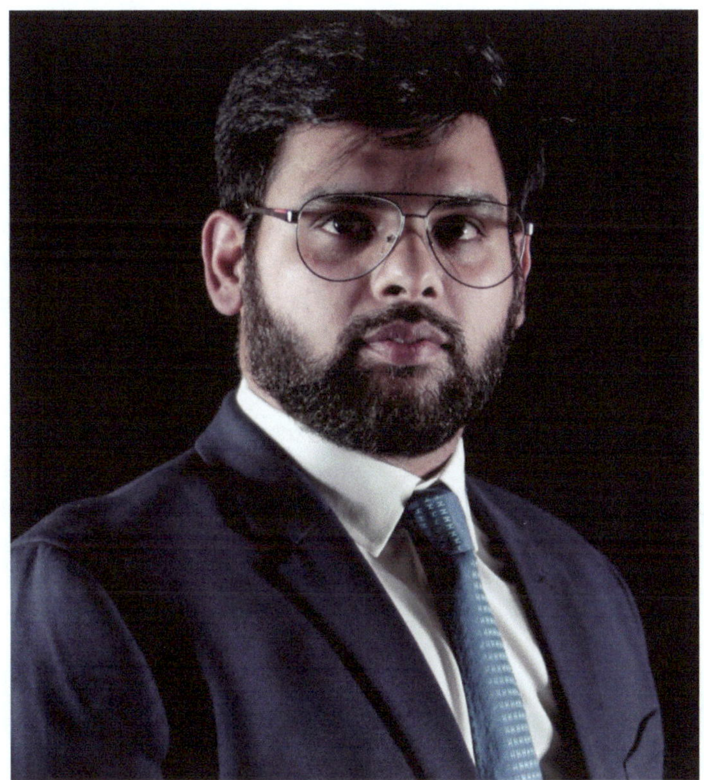

Gaurav Luthra is an accomplished author with a diverse range of experience in the medical device industry. With a career spanning 17 years, he has served as a Managing Director, leading and overseeing operations in the field. His extensive knowledge of manufacturing and new product development, regulatory affairs, quality management systems (QMS), and research and development has positioned him as an expert in his field. Throughout his career, Gaurav Luthra has contributed significantly through his research and publications. He has authored remarkable papers that have been published in renowned international journals.

As a Managing Director at KAULMED PRIVATE LIMITED (KAUL-Medizintechnik GmbH), Gaurav Luthra has been responsible for driving innovation and spearheading research and development efforts within his organization. His focus on new product development has allowed him to stay at the forefront of technological advancements in the medical device industry, ensuring that his company remains competitive and continues to provide cutting-edge solutions. In addition to his expertise in manufacturing and product development. With a holistic approach to his work, Gaurav Luthra emphasizes the importance of quality management systems. He recognizes the significance of maintaining robust processes and procedures to ensure the consistent delivery of safe and effective medical devices. Through his experience, he has implemented and optimized QMS practices to meet the highest industry standards.

Gaurav Luthra's extensive experience and comprehensive understanding of the medical device industry make him an authoritative voice in his field. His dedication to research and development, combined with his expertise in manufacturing, regulatory affairs, and QMS, positions him as a valuable resource for professionals and researchers seeking insights into the medical device industry.

As an author, Gaurav Luthra can communicate complex concepts in a clear and concise manner. Overall, Gaurav Luthra's expertise, experience, and research contributions have solidified his reputation as a prominent figure in the medical device industry. Through his publications and managerial role, he continues to make significant contributions to the advancement and improvement of medical devices, ultimately benefiting patients and healthcare providers alike.

Introduction

Regulatory compliance is of paramount importance in the healthcare industry, where adherence to laws, regulations, and guidelines is crucial for ensuring patient safety, maintaining data privacy, and promoting ethical practices. Navigating the complexities of healthcare compliance can be a daunting task for healthcare organizations, given the ever-evolving regulatory landscape and the potential consequences of non-compliance.

Regulatory compliance in the healthcare industry is a critical aspect of ensuring patient safety, maintaining data security, and adhering to ethical and legal standards. Navigating the complexities of healthcare regulations can be challenging, but it is essential for healthcare organizations to understand and comply with these requirements to avoid penalties, reputational damage, and legal issues. In this response, we'll discuss some **key aspects of regulatory compliance in the healthcare industry and provide guidance on navigating these complexities.**

1. **Know the Regulatory Landscape:** Healthcare organizations must have a comprehensive understanding of the regulatory landscape that applies to their operations. This includes familiarizing themselves with laws and regulations at the local, state, and federal levels. In the United States, key regulations include the Health Insurance Portability and Accountability Act (HIPAA), the Affordable Care Act (ACA), the Medicare Access and CHIP Reauthorization Act (MACRA), and the 21st Century Cures Act. Stay updated on changes and developments in the regulatory environment to ensure ongoing compliance.

2. **Establish Compliance Programs:** Develop robust compliance programs that align with applicable regulations and industry standards. These programs should include policies, procedures, and processes designed to ensure adherence to regulations, promote ethical behavior, and mitigate risks. Compliance programs should encompass areas such as privacy and security, billing and coding, quality improvement, and fraud prevention. Regularly review and update these programs to reflect changes in regulations and best practices.

3. **Data Privacy and Security:** Protecting patient data is a crucial aspect of regulatory compliance. Ensure compliance with privacy regulations, such as HIPAA in the United States, by implementing safeguards to secure electronic health records, establishing protocols for data breaches and incident response, and training staff on data protection best practices. Conduct regular risk assessments and audits to identify vulnerabilities and implement measures to mitigate those risks.

4. **Documentation and Record-Keeping:** Maintaining accurate and complete documentation is essential for regulatory compliance. Develop systems and processes for documenting patient care, billing, and other relevant activities. Ensure that records are securely stored, easily retrievable, and retained for the required time specified by regulations. Implement policies for proper documentation practices and educate staff on their responsibilities in record-keeping.

5. **Training and Education:** Healthcare organizations should invest in training and education programs to ensure that staff members are knowledgeable about regulatory requirements and understand their roles and responsibilities in maintaining compliance. Provide regular training on topics such as privacy and security, fraud and abuse prevention, coding and billing, and ethical conduct. Offer opportunities for ongoing education to keep staff informed about changes in regulations and emerging compliance issues.

6. **Monitoring and Auditing:** Establish a system for ongoing monitoring and auditing of compliance activities. Regularly assess adherence to policies and procedures, conduct internal audits, and implement mechanisms for reporting and addressing compliance concerns or violations. Utilize data analytics to identify trends, patterns, and potential areas of non-compliance. Implement corrective actions and continuously improve compliance efforts based on audit findings.

7. **Engage Legal and Compliance Experts:** Seek guidance from legal and compliance experts to ensure a thorough understanding of regulatory requirements and to address any compliance challenges. Consider engaging external consultants or legal counsel who specialize in healthcare compliance to provide guidance, conduct audits, and offer ongoing support in navigating regulatory complexities.

8. **Stay Informed and Adapt:** Regulatory requirements in the healthcare industry are subject to change. Stay informed about new regulations, guidance, and enforcement actions through industry publications,

professional associations, government agencies, and legal resources. Be prepared to adapt compliance programs and processes accordingly to ensure ongoing compliance.

In a nutshell, navigating regulatory compliance in the healthcare industry requires a proactive and comprehensive approach. Healthcare organizations must invest in developing robust compliance programs, prioritizing data privacy and security, maintaining accurate documentation, providing training and education to staff, monitoring compliance activities, and seeking expert guidance when needed. By doing so, organizations can navigate the complexities of regulatory compliance and uphold the highest standards of patient care, data protection, and ethical conduct in the healthcare industry.

Importance of Regulatory Compliance in the Healthcare Industry

Regulatory compliance plays a pivotal role in the healthcare industry, serving as a critical foundation for ensuring patient safety, maintaining the integrity of healthcare services, protecting sensitive information, and upholding ethical standards (Figure 1). The complex and ever-evolving nature of healthcare regulations necessitates a robust commitment to compliance from healthcare organizations. Understanding the importance of regulatory compliance in the healthcare industry is essential for all stakeholders involved, as it directly impacts the quality of care provided and the overall reputation of the organization.

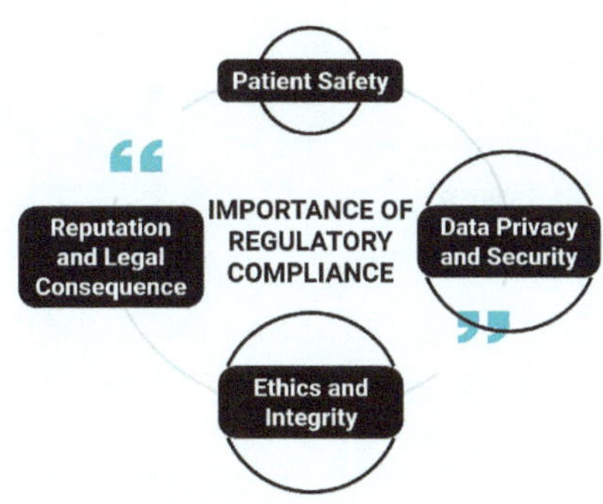

▼ **Figure 1:** Importance of Regulatory Compliance

Patient Safety:

At the core of regulatory compliance in healthcare is the fundamental principle of patient safety. Compliance with regulations helps healthcare organizations establish and maintain standards that safeguard patients from harm. Compliance programs focus on preventing medical errors, reducing adverse events, and promoting a culture of continuous improvement. By adhering to regulatory guidelines, healthcare providers can ensure that patients receive safe and effective treatments, medications, and interventions, thus minimizing the risk of harm and maximizing positive health outcomes.

Data Privacy and Security:

In an era of increasing digitalization, protecting patient information and ensuring data privacy has become paramount. Regulatory compliance, such as the Health Insurance Portability and Accountability Act (HIPAA) in the United States, sets stringent standards for the collection, use, and disclosure of patient data. Compliance with privacy and security regulations helps healthcare organizations maintain the confidentiality of patient records, prevent unauthorized access or breaches, and promote trust among patients. By safeguarding sensitive information, compliance ensures that patient privacy is respected and that personal health data is used ethically and appropriately.

Ethics and Integrity:

Healthcare organizations are entrusted with the well-being and trust of their patients. Regulatory compliance serves as a moral compass, guiding healthcare providers to uphold ethical standards in their practices. Compliance with regulations related to research ethics, patient rights, informed consent, and conflicts of interest ensures that healthcare organizations prioritize the ethical treatment of patients and maintain transparency in their operations. Compliance programs also help prevent fraud, abuse, and misconduct, fostering a culture of integrity and accountability within the healthcare industry.

Reputation and Legal Consequences:

Non-compliance with healthcare regulations can have severe consequences for organizations. Regulatory bodies and government agencies actively monitor and enforce compliance, imposing penalties, fines, and legal actions against violators. Cases of non-compliance can result in reputational damage, erosion of public trust, loss of business opportunities, and legal liabilities. On the other hand, organizations that demonstrate a commitment to regulatory compliance can enhance their reputation, attract patients, and build strong relationships with stakeholders.

Regulatory compliance is of utmost importance in the healthcare industry due to its direct impact on patient safety, data privacy, ethical practices, and organizational reputation. By adhering to regulations, healthcare organizations ensure the provision of safe and effective care, protect patient privacy, maintain ethical standards, and mitigate legal risks. Embracing a culture of compliance fosters trust among patients, employees, and stakeholders, creating a solid foundation for delivering high-quality healthcare services. In an ever-changing regulatory landscape, organizations that prioritize compliance demonstrate their commitment to ethical practices, patient well-being, and the overall advancement of the healthcare industry.

Overview of the Complexities and Challenges Faced by Healthcare Organizations

Healthcare organizations face numerous complexities and challenges that can impact their operations, patient care, and overall success. Here is an overview of some of the key complexities and challenges faced by healthcare organizations:

1. **Regulatory Compliance:** Compliance with a multitude of regulations at the local, state, and federal levels is a significant challenge for healthcare organizations. Ensuring adherence to complex regulations such as HIPAA, ACA, MACRA, and others requires significant resources and ongoing efforts to stay updated with changing requirements.

2. **Health Information Technology:** The increasing reliance on health information technology presents both opportunities and challenges. Implementing and managing electronic health records (EHRs), interoperability, data security, and privacy concerns are complex tasks. Integrating different systems and ensuring seamless data exchange between healthcare providers, payers, and other stakeholders can be challenging.

3. **Financial Pressures:** Healthcare organizations face financial challenges related to reimbursement, declining reimbursements from government and private payers, rising costs of technology and medications, and increasing overhead expenses. Balancing financial sustainability with the delivery of quality care is a constant struggle.

4. **Patient Safety and Quality Improvement:** Ensuring patient safety and delivering high-quality care are top priorities for healthcare organizations. However, achieving these goals in a complex healthcare environment with various stakeholders, evolving evidence-based practices, and the potential for human error can be challenging. Organizations must implement quality improvement initiatives, adhere to clinical guidelines, and foster a culture of safety.

5. **Workforce Shortages and Talent Management:** Healthcare organizations often face shortages of skilled healthcare professionals, including physicians, nurses, and allied health professionals. Recruiting and retaining qualified staff is challenging, particularly in rural areas and specialized fields. Additionally, managing and optimizing workforce productivity, addressing burnout, and ensuring adequate staffing levels can be complex tasks.

6. **Data Security and Privacy:** Protecting patient data from security breaches and maintaining privacy are critical challenges for healthcare organizations. With the increasing digitization of healthcare information, organizations must implement robust security measures, train staff on data protection best practices, and comply with regulations like HIPAA. The growing threat of cyberattacks and the potential for data breaches further compound these challenges.

7. **Healthcare Reform and Policy Changes:** The healthcare industry is subject to ongoing reforms and policy changes that can significantly impact operations. Changes in reimbursement models, shifts towards value-based care, and updates to healthcare regulations require healthcare organizations to adapt quickly, invest in new technologies, and implement changes in care delivery models.

8. **Interoperability and Care Coordination:** Coordinating care among multiple providers, healthcare systems, and settings is a complex challenge. Achieving interoperability between different electronic health record systems and sharing patient information securely across organizations remains a significant hurdle. Seamless care coordination is crucial for improving patient outcomes and reducing duplicative or fragmented care.

9. **Ethical and Legal Dilemmas:** Healthcare organizations often face ethical and legal dilemmas in decision-making processes. Balancing patient autonomy, confidentiality, resource allocation, and the complexities of end-of-life care can be challenging. Organizations must have ethical frameworks, policies, and committees to address these dilemmas and ensure compliance with legal and regulatory requirements.

10. **Healthcare Disparities and Access to Care:** Addressing healthcare disparities and ensuring equitable access to care are ongoing challenges for healthcare organizations. Socioeconomic factors, geographic barriers, cultural considerations, and systemic issues contribute to disparities in healthcare outcomes. Organizations must work towards improving access to care for underserved populations and reducing health inequities.

Navigating these complexities and challenges requires strategic planning, effective leadership, collaboration among stakeholders, continuous education, and a commitment to quality improvement. Healthcare organizations must adapt to the evolving landscape, leverage technology, and embrace innovative solutions to provide optimal patient care while ensuring regulatory compliance and financial sustainability.

Purpose and Scope of the Book

Purpose of the Book:

The purpose of the book "**Regulatory Compliance in the Healthcare Industry: Navigating the Complexities**" is to provide healthcare professionals, administrators, compliance officers, and other stakeholders in the healthcare sector with a comprehensive resource to understand, navigate, and address the complex landscape of regulatory compliance. The book aims to assist readers in developing effective strategies, policies, and practices to ensure compliance with the ever-changing regulatory requirements in the healthcare industry.

Scope of the Book:

The book covers a wide range of topics related to regulatory compliance in the healthcare industry. It begins with an overview of the importance of regulatory compliance and its impact on patient safety, data security, and ethical conduct. It then delves into the specific regulations that healthcare organizations need to navigate, including HIPAA, ACA, MACRA, and other relevant laws and regulations.

The scope of the book includes the following key areas:

1. **Regulatory Landscape:** Understanding the regulatory framework and its impact on healthcare organizations, including federal, state, and local regulations.

2. **Compliance Programs:** Developing and implementing comprehensive compliance programs that align with regulatory requirements and industry best practices.

3. **Data Privacy and Security:** Ensuring compliance with privacy regulations, protecting patient data, and implementing measures to prevent and respond to data breaches.

4. **Documentation and Record-Keeping:** Establishing proper documentation practices and record-keeping to meet regulatory requirements and ensure accurate and complete documentation.

5. **Training and Education:** Providing training and education to staff members on regulatory compliance, privacy, security, and ethical conduct.

6. **Monitoring and Auditing:** Establishing mechanisms for ongoing monitoring, internal audits, and corrective actions to ensure compliance with regulations.

7. **Financial Considerations:** Addressing financial pressures and reimbursement challenges while maintaining compliance with regulations.

8. **Interoperability and Technology:** Exploring the role of health information technology, interoperability, and electronic health records in regulatory compliance.

9. **Ethics and Legal Considerations:** Addressing ethical dilemmas, legal obligations, and decision-making processes in the context of regulatory compliance.

10. **Healthcare Disparities and Access to Care:** Recognizing the importance of equitable access to care and reducing healthcare disparities within the framework of regulatory compliance.

The book aims to provide practical guidance, best practices, case studies, and real-world examples to help healthcare professionals navigate the complexities of regulatory compliance effectively. It also highlights emerging trends, challenges, and future directions in the regulatory landscape to equip readers with the knowledge needed to adapt and stay compliant in an evolving healthcare environment.

Chapter 01

Understanding Regulatory Compliance

Understanding regulatory compliance involves grasping the concept, importance, and intricacies of adhering to regulations and requirements imposed by governing bodies in a specific industry (Figure 1.1). In the context of the healthcare industry, regulatory compliance refers to the adherence to laws, regulations, and guidelines set forth by governmental agencies, such as local, state, and federal authorities, as well as industry-specific regulatory bodies.

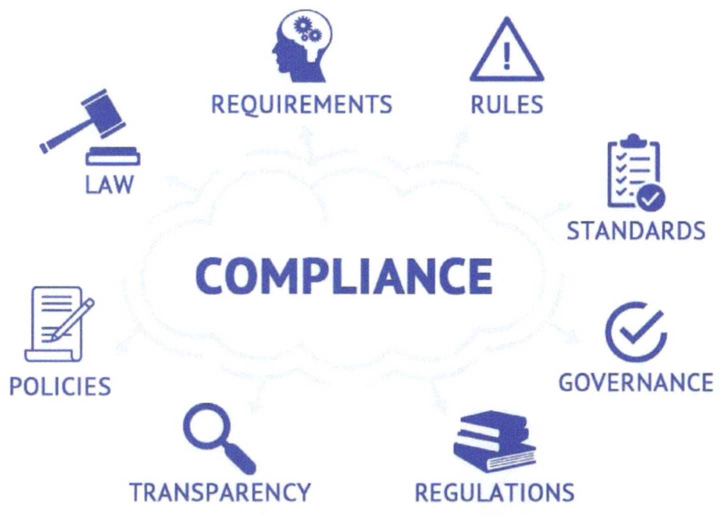

▼ **Figure 1.1:** Aspects of Understanding Regulatory Compliance

Key aspects of understanding regulatory compliance in the healthcare industry include:

1. **Laws and Regulations:** Familiarize yourself with the specific laws and regulations that apply to the healthcare industry, such as HIPAA, ACA, MACRA, and others. These regulations outline the legal requirements that healthcare organizations must comply with to ensure patient safety, data privacy, and ethical conduct.

2. **Industry Standards and Guidelines:** Apart from legal requirements, healthcare organizations often need to follow industry standards and guidelines. These standards may be established by organizations such as the Joint Commission, Centers for Medicare and Medicaid Services (CMS), or professional associations. Adhering to these standards helps ensure quality of care and best practices.

3. **Regulatory Bodies:** Identify the regulatory bodies responsible for overseeing compliance in the healthcare industry. These may include federal agencies like the Office for Civil Rights (OCR) and the Centers for Medicare and Medicaid Services (CMS), as well as state health departments and local governing bodies. Understand their roles, responsibilities, and enforcement mechanisms.

4. **Compliance Programs:** Implementing a comprehensive compliance program is essential. It should include policies, procedures, and processes designed to ensure adherence to regulations and mitigate risks. Compliance programs should address areas such as privacy and security, billing and coding, quality improvement, and fraud prevention.

5. **Risk Assessment and Management:** Conduct regular risk assessments to identify potential compliance risks and vulnerabilities within your organization. Implement risk management strategies and controls to mitigate these risks effectively. This may involve measures like regular audits, training programs, and monitoring mechanisms.

6. **Training and Education:** Provide ongoing training and education to employees to ensure they understand their roles and responsibilities in compliance. Training should cover topics such as privacy and security, coding and billing, fraud and abuse prevention, and ethical conduct. Regularly update training programs to reflect changes in regulations and emerging compliance issues.

7. **Documentation and Record-Keeping:** Accurate and thorough documentation is crucial for compliance. Develop systems and processes for documenting patient care, billing, and other relevant activities. Ensure records are securely stored, easily retrievable, and retained for the required time specified by regulations.

8. **Monitoring and Auditing:** Regularly monitor and audit compliance activities within your organization. This includes internal audits, self-assessments, and ongoing monitoring of policies and procedures. Establish mechanisms for reporting and addressing compliance concerns or violations.

9. **Enforcement and Consequences:** Understand the potential consequences of non-compliance, including penalties, fines, legal actions, reputational damage, and exclusion from government programs. Stay informed about enforcement actions and cases related to regulatory compliance in the healthcare industry.

10. **Staying Up to Date:** Stay current with regulatory changes, updates, and emerging trends. Regularly review resources, publications, and updates from regulatory bodies, industry associations, and professional networks. Engage with legal and compliance experts to seek guidance and stay informed about the evolving regulatory landscape.

By understanding regulatory compliance, healthcare organizations can navigate the complexities, mitigate risks, and maintain the highest standards of patient care, data security, and ethical conduct in the healthcare industry.

Definition and Significance of Regulatory Compliance in Healthcare

Definition of Regulatory Compliance in Healthcare:

Regulatory compliance in healthcare refers to the adherence and conformity of healthcare organizations, providers, and professionals to the laws, regulations, guidelines, and standards set by governing bodies at local, state, and federal levels. It encompasses meeting the legal and ethical obligations imposed by regulatory authorities to ensure patient safety, protect data privacy, maintain quality of care, and promote ethical conduct within the healthcare industry.

Significance of Regulatory Compliance in Healthcare:

Regulatory compliance holds significant importance in the healthcare industry for several reasons:

1. **Patient Safety:** Compliance with regulations helps safeguard patient safety by ensuring that healthcare organizations maintain high standards of care delivery, infection control, medication management, and other critical areas that impact patient well-being.

2. **Data Privacy and Security:** Regulatory compliance, such as adherence to the Health Insurance Portability and Accountability Act (HIPAA), safeguards

patient data privacy and ensures secure handling of electronic health records (EHRs) to protect against data breaches and unauthorized access.

3. **Legal and Ethical Obligations:** Compliance with healthcare regulations ensures that organizations and professionals uphold legal and ethical standards, promoting transparency, integrity, and ethical conduct in their interactions with patients, colleagues, and other stakeholders.

4. **Quality of Care:** Regulatory compliance often involves adherence to industry standards and guidelines, which focus on maintaining and improving the quality of care provided. Compliance programs and standards support the adoption of evidence-based practices and promote continuous quality improvement.

5. **Reputation and Trust:** Demonstrating compliance with healthcare regulations enhances the reputation and trust of healthcare organizations and professionals. Compliance instills confidence in patients, insurers, and regulatory bodies, and contributes to the overall credibility of the healthcare organization.

6. **Avoiding Penalties and Legal Consequences:** Non-compliance with healthcare regulations can result in penalties, fines, legal actions, loss of licensure, or exclusion from government programs, which can have severe financial and reputational consequences for organizations and individuals.

7. **Risk Mitigation:** Compliance programs help identify and mitigate risks associated with legal, operational, and financial aspects of healthcare operations. Through risk assessments, audits, and monitoring, compliance efforts help identify vulnerabilities and implement measures to minimize potential risks.

8. **Data Sharing and Interoperability:** Compliance with regulatory requirements supports the seamless exchange of patient information and interoperability between healthcare systems, enabling better care coordination and improving patient outcomes.

9. **Alignment with Best Practices:** Healthcare regulations often incorporate industry best practices, evidence-based guidelines, and standards developed by regulatory bodies and professional associations. Compliance ensures alignment with these practices, which can enhance efficiency, effectiveness, and patient outcomes.

10. **Adapting to Regulatory Changes:** Regulatory compliance requires healthcare organizations to stay updated with evolving regulations and

adapt their practices accordingly. This helps organizations remain current with the latest legal requirements, industry trends, and emerging challenges in healthcare.

Overall, regulatory compliance is essential for healthcare organizations to fulfill their responsibilities, protect patients, maintain data security and privacy, uphold ethical standards, and operate within the legal framework. It promotes patient safety, quality care, and ethical conduct while mitigating risks and ensuring accountability within the healthcare industry.

Key Regulatory Bodies and Their Roles (FDA, CMS, HIPAA, etc.)

Several key regulatory bodies play crucial roles in the healthcare industry, each with specific responsibilities and jurisdictions. Here are some of the prominent regulatory bodies and their roles:

1. **Food and Drug Administration (FDA):** The FDA is a federal agency responsible for protecting public health by ensuring the safety, efficacy, and security of drugs, medical devices, vaccines, biologics, and food products. The FDA regulates the development, manufacturing, labeling, and marketing of these products, conducting inspections and enforcing regulations to maintain safety and quality standards.

2. **Centers for Medicare and Medicaid Services (CMS):** CMS is a federal agency within the U.S. Department of Health and Human Services (HHS) that administers Medicare, Medicaid, and other healthcare programs. CMS oversees reimbursement policies, manages quality improvement initiatives, and enforces regulations to ensure program integrity and proper billing practices.

3. **Office for Civil Rights (OCR):** OCR is a division of the U.S. Department of Health and Human Services (HHS) responsible for enforcing compliance with the Health Insurance Portability and Accountability Act (HIPAA). OCR ensures the protection of individuals' health information privacy rights and investigates complaints related to HIPAA violations.

4. **Centers for Disease Control and Prevention (CDC):** The CDC is a federal agency focused on protecting public health and safety. It provides guidance and conducts research to prevent and control infectious diseases, manages public health emergencies, promotes health promotion and prevention

efforts, and issues guidelines and recommendations for healthcare providers.

5. **Occupational Safety and Health Administration (OSHA):** OSHA is a federal agency responsible for ensuring safe and healthy working conditions for employees in various industries, including healthcare. OSHA sets standards, conducts inspections, and enforces regulations related to occupational safety, including hazard communication, blood-borne pathogens, and workplace violence prevention.

6. **National Institutes of Health (NIH):** NIH is the primary agency of the United States government responsible for biomedical and public health research. It provides funding for research grants, conducts medical research, and supports scientific advancements to improve human health and address various diseases and conditions.

7. **Drug Enforcement Administration (DEA):** The DEA is a federal agency under the U.S. Department of Justice that enforces controlled substances laws and regulations. It regulates the manufacturing, distribution, dispensing, and prescribing of controlled substances, including prescription medications, to prevent their misuse and abuse.

8. **State Health Departments:** Each state has its own health department responsible for implementing and enforcing state-specific health regulations and overseeing public health initiatives. State health departments may have additional roles in licensing healthcare facilities, conducting inspections, and addressing health emergencies.

These regulatory bodies work together to ensure the safety, quality, and ethical standards within the healthcare industry. They establish and enforce regulations, conduct inspections, provide guidance, and take enforcement actions to protect public health, patient safety, and data privacy. Healthcare organizations must understand the roles and responsibilities of these regulatory bodies to comply with the relevant regulations and requirements.

Impact of Non-compliance on Healthcare Organizations

Non-compliance with healthcare regulations can have significant impacts on healthcare organizations, affecting their operations, financial stability, reputation, and legal standing. Here are some key impacts of non-compliance (Figure 1.2):

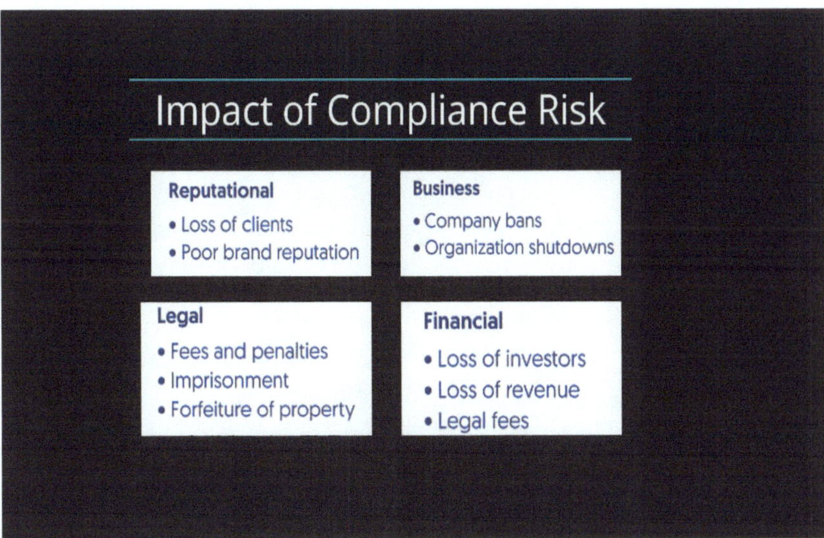

▼ **Figure 1.2:** Impact of Compliance Risk

1. **Financial Consequences:** Non-compliance can result in financial penalties, fines, and legal settlements. These financial burdens can significantly strain the resources of healthcare organizations, affecting their profitability and ability to provide quality care.

2. **Loss of Reimbursements:** Non-compliance with regulations, such as those related to coding, billing, and documentation, may lead to denied or reduced reimbursements from government payers, private insurers, and Medicare/Medicaid programs. This loss of revenue can impact the financial viability of healthcare organizations.

3. **Legal Actions and Litigation:** Non-compliance can result in legal actions, including lawsuits, investigations, and regulatory audits. Legal proceedings can be costly and time-consuming, leading to reputational damage and potential monetary damages.

4. **Reputational Damage:** Non-compliance can tarnish the reputation of healthcare organizations. Negative publicity, media attention, and public perception of non-compliance can erode trust among patients, insurers, and the community. Rebuilding trust and regaining a positive reputation can be challenging.

5. **Exclusion from Government Programs:** Non-compliance with healthcare regulations may result in exclusion from participation in government programs such as Medicare, Medicaid, or other federal healthcare

initiatives. This exclusion can have severe consequences, limiting the organization's patient base and access to funding.

6. **Compromised Patient Safety and Quality of Care:** Non-compliance with regulations related to patient safety, infection control, and quality of care can directly impact patient outcomes. Failure to meet standards and guidelines may result in medical errors, compromised patient safety, and substandard care, leading to adverse events and poor clinical outcomes.

7. **Data Breaches and Privacy Violations:** Non-compliance with data privacy and security regulations, such as HIPAA, can lead to data breaches and privacy violations. This can result in significant reputational damage, loss of patient trust, regulatory investigations, and potential legal actions.

8. **Operational Disruptions and Remediation Costs:** Non-compliance often necessitates corrective actions and remediation efforts, such as process changes, staff retraining, implementing new systems, and enhancing infrastructure. These operational disruptions and associated costs can strain the resources and productivity of healthcare organizations.

9. **Loss of Licensure and Accreditation:** Persistent non-compliance with regulatory requirements can lead to the loss of licensure or accreditation, making it difficult to operate legally and limiting the organization's ability to provide services or access certain markets.

10. **Impact on Staff Morale and Retention:** Non-compliance issues can create an environment of uncertainty, stress, and mistrust among staff members. This can negatively affect morale, employee retention, and overall organizational culture.

It is essential for healthcare organizations to prioritize regulatory compliance to avoid these detrimental impacts. By investing in compliance programs, continuous education, and robust processes, healthcare organizations can mitigate the risks associated with non-compliance and maintain their commitment to patient safety, quality care, and ethical conduct.

Emerging Trends and Developments in Healthcare Regulations

Emerging trends and developments in healthcare regulations reflect the evolving landscape of the industry, technological advancements, changing patient needs, and policy priorities (Figure 1.3). Here are some key trends and developments in healthcare regulations:

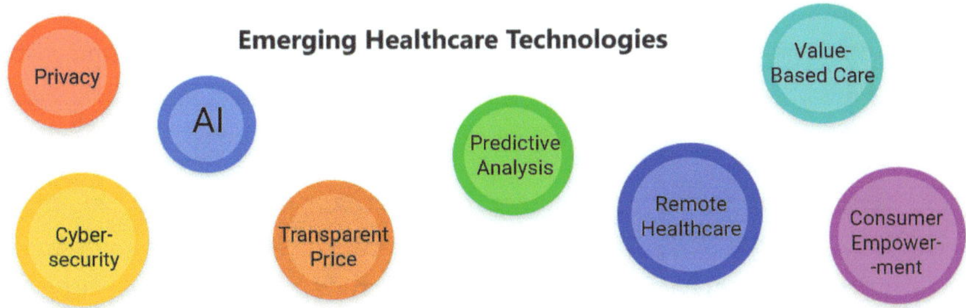

▼ **Figure 1.3: Benefits of Healthcare Technology**

1. **Digital Health and Telemedicine:** The rapid growth of digital health technologies and telemedicine has prompted the need for updated regulations. Regulatory bodies are addressing issues such as licensure, privacy and security, reimbursement, and the use of virtual care platforms to ensure safe and effective delivery of healthcare services.

2. **Data Privacy and Security:** With the increasing digitization of healthcare data, there is a growing focus on strengthening data privacy and security regulations. Governments and regulatory bodies are enacting stricter regulations to protect patient information, address data breaches, and enforce penalties for non-compliance, such as the European Union's General Data Protection Regulation (GDPR).

3. **Interoperability and Health Information Exchange:** There is a push for improved interoperability and seamless health information exchange between different healthcare systems, providers, and stakeholders. Regulatory initiatives, such as the 21st Century Cures Act and Fast Healthcare Interoperability Resources (FHIR) standards, aim to facilitate data sharing and enhance care coordination.

4. **Value-Based Care and Alternative Payment Models:** The shift towards value-based care and alternative payment models is transforming reimbursement and regulatory frameworks. Regulations are being revised to incentivize quality outcomes, care coordination, and cost containment, such as the Medicare Access and CHIP Reauthorization Act (MACRA) and bundled payment initiatives.

5. **Cybersecurity and Data Breach Notification:** With the rising threat of cyberattacks and data breaches in healthcare, regulations are being strengthened to address cybersecurity vulnerabilities. This includes

requirements for organizations to implement robust security measures, conduct risk assessments, and develop incident response plans. Additionally, regulations are mandating prompt notification and disclosure of data breaches to affected individuals and regulatory bodies.

6. **Drug Pricing and Transparency:** Rising drug costs have led to increased scrutiny and the implementation of regulations aimed at promoting drug pricing transparency. Regulatory efforts are focusing on enhancing price transparency, requiring manufacturers to disclose drug prices, and addressing pharmaceutical industry practices that may impact drug affordability and access.

7. **Health Equity and Social Determinants of Health:** There is a growing recognition of health disparities and the impact of social determinants of health on population health outcomes. Regulatory efforts are aiming to address health equity by promoting access to care, addressing disparities, and integrating social determinants of health into care delivery and payment models.

8. **Artificial Intelligence (AI) and Machine Learning:** The use of AI and machine learning in healthcare is driving the need for regulatory frameworks to address issues such as algorithm transparency, data bias, patient privacy, and the ethical use of AI technologies. Regulatory bodies are developing guidelines and policies to ensure safe and responsible integration of AI in healthcare.

9. **Opioid Crisis and Substance Abuse:** The opioid crisis has prompted regulatory responses to address opioid prescribing practices, improve prescription drug monitoring programs, expand access to addiction treatment services, and enhance regulations related to controlled substances. Efforts are focused on balancing pain management needs with strategies to combat substance abuse.

10. **Consumer Empowerment and Patient Rights:** Regulatory initiatives are aimed at empowering patients, enhancing transparency, and ensuring patient rights. This includes regulations related to informed consent, access to health records, patient engagement, and the right to choose healthcare providers.

These emerging trends and developments in healthcare regulations reflect the ongoing efforts to adapt regulatory frameworks to address the evolving healthcare landscape, technological advancements, patient needs, and policy priorities. Healthcare organizations must stay informed about these developments to ensure compliance, adapt their practices, and provide high-quality, patient-centered care in a rapidly changing regulatory environment.

Building a Compliance Program

Building a compliance program is an essential undertaking for healthcare organizations to uphold ethical standards, mitigate risks, and ensure adherence to regulatory requirements. The process begins with establishing clear compliance governance and assigning dedicated compliance officers or teams. A thorough risk assessment helps identify potential compliance vulnerabilities. Developing comprehensive policies and procedures tailored to the organization's specific operations is crucial. Equally important is providing robust training and education programs to staff members to ensure their understanding of compliance requirements and their role in maintaining compliance. Implementing internal controls, monitoring mechanisms, and reporting channels foster a culture of transparency and accountability. Regular audits and reviews help assess program effectiveness and identify areas for improvement. Keeping abreast of regulatory changes and engaging legal and compliance experts provide guidance in navigating complexities. By following these steps, healthcare organizations can build a strong compliance program that promotes ethical conduct, mitigates risks, and ensures adherence to regulatory standards (Figure 2.1).

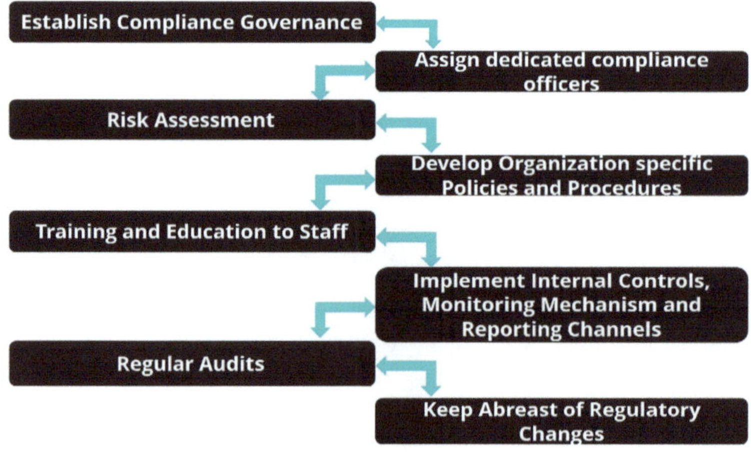

▼ **Figure 2.1:** Flowchart Representing Building of a Compliance Program

Building a robust compliance program is crucial for healthcare organizations to ensure adherence to regulatory requirements, mitigate risks, and promote ethical conduct. Here are the key steps involved in building an effective compliance program:

1. **Establish Compliance Governance:** Start by assigning clear roles and responsibilities for compliance within the organization. Designate a compliance officer or team responsible for overseeing and managing the compliance program. Ensure they have the necessary authority and resources to carry out their responsibilities effectively.

2. **Conduct a Risk Assessment:** Perform a comprehensive risk assessment to identify potential compliance risks and vulnerabilities within the organization. This assessment should cover areas such as privacy and security, billing and coding, quality improvement, fraud prevention, and other relevant regulatory domains. Identify potential risks and prioritize them based on their potential impact and likelihood of occurrence.

3. **Develop Policies and Procedures:** Develop a set of policies and procedures that outline the organization's commitment to compliance, as well as specific guidelines for various regulatory requirements. Policies should be tailored to the organization's specific operations and reflect applicable laws and regulations. Ensure that policies are easily accessible, clearly communicated to staff, and regularly updated to reflect changes in regulations.

4. **Training and Education:** Provide comprehensive training and education programs to staff members to ensure their understanding of compliance requirements and their roles in maintaining compliance. Training should cover topics such as privacy and security, fraud prevention, coding and billing, and ethical conduct. Regularly update training programs to address new regulations and emerging compliance issues.

5. **Implement Internal Controls and Monitoring:** Establish internal controls and monitoring mechanisms to detect and prevent compliance violations. This may include routine audits, self-assessments, and periodic reviews of operations and processes. Implement monitoring tools, such as data analytics, to identify patterns, trends, and potential areas of non-compliance. Develop processes for reporting and addressing compliance concerns or violations.

6. **Encourage Reporting and Non-Retaliation:** Create a culture that encourages employees to report compliance concerns or potential violations without fear of retaliation. Implement mechanisms for anonymous reporting and provide clear channels for reporting concerns, such as a confidential hotline or reporting system. Establish a non-retaliation policy to protect employees who report compliance issues in good faith.

7. **Enforce Disciplinary Actions:** Develop a system for enforcing disciplinary actions in cases of compliance violations. Clearly communicate the consequences of non-compliance, including disciplinary measures, up to and including termination of employment, where appropriate. Ensure consistency in the application of disciplinary actions to promote fairness and deter non-compliant behavior.

8. **Periodic Audits and Reviews:** Conduct regular internal audits and reviews to assess the effectiveness of the compliance program. Evaluate the organization's adherence to policies and procedures, identify areas for improvement, and implement corrective actions as necessary. Engage external consultants or legal counsel for independent audits or assessments, if needed.

9. **Keep Abreast of Regulatory Changes:** Stay updated with changes in regulations, guidance, and enforcement actions. Regularly review resources, publications, and updates from regulatory bodies, industry associations, and legal resources. Engage legal and compliance experts to seek guidance on navigating regulatory complexities and ensuring ongoing compliance.

10. **Promote a Culture of Compliance:** Foster a culture of compliance throughout the organization by promoting ethical conduct, transparency, and accountability. Ensure that compliance is integrated into the organization's values, mission, and decision-making processes. Communicate the importance of compliance to all stakeholders, including leadership, staff members, and business partners.

Building a compliance program is an ongoing process that requires continuous monitoring, evaluation, and adaptation to changing regulatory requirements. By following these steps, healthcare organizations can establish a strong compliance program that promotes ethical behavior, mitigates risks, and ensures adherence to regulatory standards.

The Essential Components of a Robust Compliance Program

A robust compliance program encompasses several essential components that work together to ensure adherence to regulatory requirements and promote ethical behavior within a healthcare organization. Here are the key components of a robust compliance program:

1. **Compliance Policies and Procedures:** Clearly defined and comprehensive policies and procedures outline the organization's commitment to compliance. These documents provide guidance to employees on expected behaviors, regulatory requirements, and specific compliance areas such as privacy and security, billing and coding, and ethical conduct.

2. **Compliance Officer or Team:** Assigning a dedicated compliance officer or team responsible for overseeing the compliance program is crucial. They should have the necessary expertise, authority, and resources to implement and manage compliance efforts effectively. The compliance officer acts as a central point of contact for compliance-related matters.

3. **Risk Assessment and Management:** Conducting regular risk assessments helps identify potential compliance risks and vulnerabilities within the organization. Assessments should cover various regulatory domains and prioritize risks based on their potential impact and likelihood. Risk management strategies and controls are then implemented to mitigate identified risks.

4. **Training and Education:** Comprehensive training and education programs ensure that employees understand their compliance obligations and responsibilities. Training should cover relevant laws and regulations, policies and procedures, privacy and security, fraud prevention, and ethical conduct. Regular updates and refresher training sessions keep employees informed about changing regulations and emerging compliance issues.

5. **Internal Controls and Monitoring:** Establishing internal controls and monitoring mechanisms helps detect and prevent compliance violations. This includes conducting regular audits, self-assessments, and reviews of operations and processes. Monitoring tools such as data analytics can be employed to identify patterns, trends, and potential areas of non-compliance. Reporting

channels are put in place for employees to report compliance concerns or potential violations.

6. **Enforcement and Disciplinary Actions:** Clearly defined disciplinary actions demonstrate the organization's commitment to compliance. A system for enforcing disciplinary measures in cases of non-compliance should be implemented. This ensures consistency in addressing compliance violations and acts as a deterrent against future non-compliant behavior.

7. **Oversight and Accountability:** Senior leadership and the governing body play a crucial role in providing oversight and accountability for the compliance program. They should actively support and promote a culture of compliance, allocate resources, and regularly review the effectiveness of the program. The compliance officer reports directly to leadership and provides regular updates on compliance activities.

8. **Continuous Improvement:** A robust compliance program includes a commitment to continuous improvement. Regular assessments, evaluations, and audits help identify areas for improvement and drive the implementation of corrective actions. The program should evolve alongside changing regulatory requirements, industry best practices, and emerging risks.

9. **Documentation and Record-Keeping:** Maintaining accurate and detailed documentation is vital to demonstrate compliance efforts. Documentation includes policies and procedures, training records, risk assessments, audit findings, corrective actions, and any other relevant compliance-related documentation. Proper record-keeping ensures transparency, supports audits and investigations, and demonstrates the organization's commitment to compliance.

10. **Monitoring Regulatory Changes:** Staying up to date with regulatory changes is critical for maintaining compliance. Regularly reviewing updates, guidance, and enforcement actions from regulatory bodies helps ensure that the compliance program aligns with the most current requirements. Engaging legal and compliance experts can provide guidance on interpreting and implementing regulatory changes effectively.

By integrating these essential components into a compliance program, healthcare organizations can establish a robust framework that promotes ethical behavior, reduces risks, ensures adherence to regulatory standards, and fosters a culture of compliance throughout the organization.

Creating a Culture of Compliance within the Organization

Creating a culture of compliance within an organization is crucial for promoting ethical behavior, fostering accountability, and ensuring adherence to regulatory requirements. Here are key steps to foster a culture of compliance:

1. **Leadership Commitment:** Demonstrate visible and unwavering commitment to compliance from the top leadership of the organization. Leaders should actively communicate the importance of compliance, allocate necessary resources, and lead by example in ethical decision-making and conduct.

2. **Clear Expectations and Policies:** Clearly communicate expectations regarding compliance through comprehensive policies and procedures. Ensure that policies are easily accessible, easily understood, and consistently enforced. Reinforce the message that compliance is a fundamental aspect of the organization's values and mission.

3. **Training and Education:** Provide regular and comprehensive training programs to educate employees about their compliance obligations and the organization's commitment to ethical conduct. Offer training on topics such as regulatory requirements, privacy and security, fraud prevention, and ethical decision-making.

4. **Open Communication Channels:** Establish channels for employees to ask questions, seek guidance, and report compliance concerns without fear of retaliation. Encourage an open-door policy and maintain confidentiality in the reporting process. Regularly communicate updates, changes in regulations, and compliance-related information to all employees.

5. **Lead by Example:** Leaders and managers should exemplify ethical behavior and compliance in their own actions. This includes following policies, engaging in transparent and ethical decision-making, and maintaining high standards of conduct. When employees see their leaders prioritizing compliance, it reinforces the importance of compliance throughout the organization.

6. **Accountability and Disciplinary Actions:** Implement a consistent and fair disciplinary process for non-compliance. Ensure that violations are promptly and appropriately addressed, and disciplinary actions are consistently applied. Reinforce the message that compliance is non-negotiable, and violations will not be tolerated.

7. **Reward Ethical Behavior:** Recognize and reward employees who consistently demonstrate ethical behavior and compliance. Acknowledge individuals or teams that go above and beyond in upholding compliance standards. This reinforces the positive aspects of compliance and encourages others to follow suit.

8. **Continuous Monitoring and Improvement:** Regularly assess and monitor the effectiveness of the compliance program. This includes conducting internal audits, assessments, and reviews to identify areas for improvement. Solicit feedback from employees regarding compliance challenges or suggestions for enhancing the program. Use the insights gained to refine and strengthen the compliance culture.

9. **Promote Transparency and Reporting:** Encourage a transparent environment where employees feel comfortable reporting potential compliance issues. Establish anonymous reporting mechanisms, such as hotlines or reporting systems, to protect individuals who raise concerns in good faith. Actively address reported concerns and communicate the actions taken to resolve them.

10. **Embed Compliance in Performance Evaluation:** Integrate compliance expectations into performance evaluations and recognition programs. Reward and recognize employees who consistently demonstrate ethical behavior and compliance. Incorporate compliance metrics into performance goals to emphasize its importance.

By following these steps, healthcare organizations can foster a culture of compliance where ethical behavior and adherence to regulations are valued and ingrained in the organization's DNA. A strong culture of compliance helps mitigate risks, enhance patient safety, protect data privacy, and maintain the organization's reputation and integrity.

Role of Compliance Officers and their Responsibilities

The role of compliance officers in healthcare organizations is crucial for establishing and maintaining a robust compliance program. Compliance officers are responsible for ensuring adherence to laws, regulations, and ethical standards within the organization. Here are some key responsibilities of compliance officers:

1. **Developing and Implementing Compliance Programs:** Compliance officers are responsible for developing, implementing, and managing compliance

programs tailored to the organization's specific needs and regulatory requirements. This involves creating policies, procedures, and guidelines to ensure compliance with applicable laws and regulations.

2. **Monitoring and Assessing Compliance:** Compliance officers monitor the organization's compliance with laws, regulations, and internal policies. They conduct periodic risk assessments, internal audits, and compliance reviews to identify potential compliance vulnerabilities, gaps, and risks.

3. **Providing Guidance and Training:** Compliance officers provide guidance and training to employees at all levels of the organization. They educate staff members on compliance policies, regulations, and best practices, ensuring a clear understanding of their roles and responsibilities in maintaining compliance.

4. **Responding to Compliance Concerns and Violations:** Compliance officers establish mechanisms for reporting compliance concerns and potential violations, such as anonymous hotlines or reporting systems. They investigate reported concerns, respond to compliance incidents, and take appropriate corrective actions to address non-compliance.

5. **Keeping Abreast of Regulatory Changes:** Compliance officers stay informed about changes in laws, regulations, and industry standards that affect the organization. They continuously monitor regulatory updates and assess the impact on the organization's compliance program, ensuring necessary adjustments are made to maintain compliance.

6. **Collaborating with Regulatory Bodies:** Compliance officers interact with regulatory bodies, such as government agencies and accrediting organizations. They engage in communications, respond to inquiries, and provide necessary documentation during regulatory audits or investigations.

7. **Promoting a Culture of Compliance:** Compliance officers play a vital role in fostering a culture of compliance within the organization. They promote ethical behavior, transparency, and accountability, ensuring that compliance is integrated into the organization's values, mission, and decision-making processes.

8. **Providing Compliance Reporting and Documentation:** Compliance officers compile and maintain documentation related to the organization's compliance efforts. They generate compliance reports, document audit findings, and provide regular updates to senior management and the board of directors on the status of the compliance program.

9. **Staying Current with Industry Trends and Best Practices:** Compliance officers continuously educate themselves on emerging trends, industry best practices, and evolving compliance requirements. They engage in professional development activities and participate in relevant industry conferences and networks to stay up to date.

10. **Risk Management and Mitigation:** Compliance officers play a role in risk management by identifying potential compliance risks and implementing measures to mitigate them. They collaborate with other departments to ensure that compliance is integrated into strategic planning and operational decision-making.

Overall, compliance officers are responsible for establishing a culture of compliance, developing and implementing compliance programs, monitoring adherence to regulations, responding to compliance concerns, and ensuring ongoing compliance within healthcare organizations. They serve as the organization's internal regulatory and ethical compass, promoting integrity, accountability, and the delivery of high-quality care in compliance with applicable laws and regulations.

Establishing Policies, Procedures, and Internal Controls

Establishing clear policies, procedures, and internal controls is vital for healthcare organizations to ensure compliance with regulations, mitigate risks, and promote consistent practices. Here are the key components involved in establishing these elements:

1. **Policies:** Policies are high-level statements that outline the organization's commitment to compliance and provide guidance on expected behaviors and actions. When establishing policies, consider areas such as privacy and security, billing and coding, ethical conduct, quality improvement, and fraud prevention. Policies should align with relevant laws, regulations, and industry standards.

2. **Procedures:** Procedures provide step-by-step instructions on how to implement policies and achieve compliance goals. They are more detailed and specific than policies and serve as a practical guide for employees to follow. Procedures should cover areas such as patient consent, data breach response, incident reporting, coding and billing practices, and documentation requirements.

3. **Internal Controls:** Internal controls are mechanisms put in place to prevent, detect, and correct compliance violations. They are designed to ensure that processes and activities are carried out in accordance with established policies and procedures. Internal controls may include segregation of duties, authorization processes, documentation requirements, checks and balances, and regular reviews.

4. **Risk Assessment:** Conduct a comprehensive risk assessment to identify potential compliance risks and vulnerabilities within the organization. This assessment involves analyzing processes, systems, and activities to identify areas where compliance breaches are more likely to occur. The findings from the risk assessment can inform the development of policies, procedures, and internal controls.

5. **Stakeholder Involvement:** Involve relevant stakeholders, such as compliance officers, legal counsel, department heads, and frontline staff, in the development of policies, procedures, and internal controls. Their input ensures that the established frameworks are practical, realistic, and aligned with the organization's operations and goals. Seek feedback and collaboration throughout the process.

6. **Documentation:** Document all policies, procedures, and internal controls in a clear and accessible manner. Ensure that they are easily understandable by staff members and readily available for reference. Document updates, revisions, and version control to maintain a record of changes made to policies and procedures over time.

7. **Communication and Training:** Communicate the policies, procedures, and internal controls effectively to all relevant staff members. Provide training sessions, workshops, or online modules to educate employees on their roles and responsibilities in adhering to the established frameworks. Regularly reinforce compliance expectations through ongoing communication channels.

8. **Review and Updates:** Regularly review and update policies, procedures, and internal controls to reflect changes in regulations, industry best practices, and organizational needs. Stay vigilant for emerging compliance risks and address them promptly. Periodically assess the effectiveness of the established frameworks and make adjustments as necessary.

9. **Compliance Oversight:** Establish mechanisms for ongoing compliance oversight, such as internal audits, monitoring, and reporting. Assign responsibility for monitoring adherence to policies and procedures,

identifying potential compliance gaps, and reporting any issues to the compliance officer or relevant stakeholders.

10. **Continuous Improvement:** Foster a culture of continuous improvement by encouraging feedback, learning from incidents or near misses, and implementing corrective actions. Regularly assess the effectiveness of policies, procedures, and internal controls, seeking input from staff members and stakeholders for potential enhancements.

By establishing clear policies, procedures, and internal controls, healthcare organizations can provide guidelines for compliance, mitigate risks, and ensure consistent practices throughout the organization. These elements lay the foundation for effective compliance management and support a culture of integrity and accountability.

Conducting Risk Assessments and Implementing Risk Management Strategies

Conducting risk assessments and implementing risk management strategies are crucial steps in maintaining a robust compliance program within healthcare organizations. Here are the key components involved in conducting risk assessments and implementing risk management strategies (Figure 2.2):

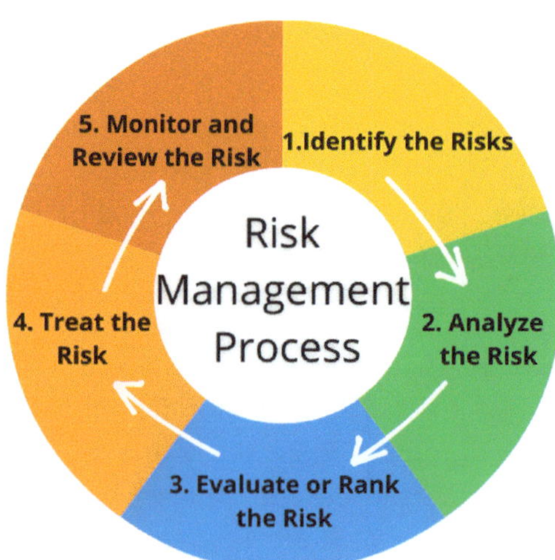

▼ **Figure 2.2:** Overview of Risk Management Process

1. **Identify and Define Risks:** Identify and define potential risks that may impact the organization's compliance efforts. This includes risks related to regulatory compliance, patient safety, data privacy and security, fraud, billing and coding, and other areas specific to the healthcare industry.

2. **Assess Risks:** Evaluate the likelihood and potential impact of each identified risk. Consider factors such as the probability of occurrence, severity of consequences, and any existing controls or mitigation measures in place. Prioritize risks based on their significance and potential impact on the organization.

3. **Risk Analysis and Evaluation:** Conduct a thorough analysis of each identified risk, examining its causes, contributing factors, and potential consequences. Evaluate the effectiveness of existing controls and mitigation strategies in managing the risks. Determine the organization's tolerance for each risk based on its strategic objectives and risk appetite.

4. **Develop Risk Management Strategies:** Develop risk management strategies and action plans to address the identified risks. This may involve implementing additional controls, modifying existing processes, enhancing training and education programs, or establishing new policies and procedures. Ensure that risk management strategies align with regulatory requirements and industry best practices.

5. **Implement Risk Controls and Mitigation Measures:** Implement risk controls and mitigation measures to reduce the likelihood or impact of identified risks. This may include segregation of duties, process redesign, enhancing data privacy and security measures, conducting regular audits and monitoring activities, and establishing reporting mechanisms for compliance concerns.

6. **Assign Responsibility and Accountability:** Clearly assign responsibility and accountability for each risk management strategy or action plan. Identify individuals or teams responsible for implementing and monitoring risk controls. Establish reporting mechanisms to track progress and ensure ongoing compliance with risk management strategies.

7. **Monitor and Review:** Continuously monitor and review the effectiveness of implemented risk controls and mitigation measures. Regularly assess and update the risk management strategies based on changes in regulations, industry trends, and organizational needs. Conduct periodic reviews and audits to evaluate the performance of risk management efforts.

8. **Communication and Training:** Communicate risk management strategies and expectations to employees at all levels of the organization. Provide training and education programs to ensure understanding and compliance with risk controls and mitigation measures. Foster a culture of risk awareness and accountability throughout the organization.

9. **Continuous Improvement:** Foster a culture of continuous improvement by encouraging feedback and learning from risk incidents or near misses. Analyze the effectiveness of risk management strategies, identify areas for improvement, and implement corrective actions as necessary. Regularly reassess risks and update risk management strategies accordingly.

10. **Documentation and Reporting:** Maintain documentation of risk assessments, risk management strategies, and associated actions taken. Keep records of ongoing monitoring, reviews, and any changes made to risk management efforts. Establish reporting mechanisms to communicate risk status, incidents, and mitigation measures to relevant stakeholders.

By conducting thorough risk assessments and implementing effective risk management strategies, healthcare organizations can proactively identify and address potential compliance risks. This promotes a culture of risk awareness, strengthens the compliance program, and enhances the organization's ability to meet regulatory requirements and maintain patient safety and data privacy.

Healthcare Privacy and Security Regulations

Healthcare privacy and security regulations are critical for safeguarding patient information, ensuring data confidentiality, and protecting individuals' privacy rights. Here are some key healthcare privacy and security regulations (Figure 3.1):

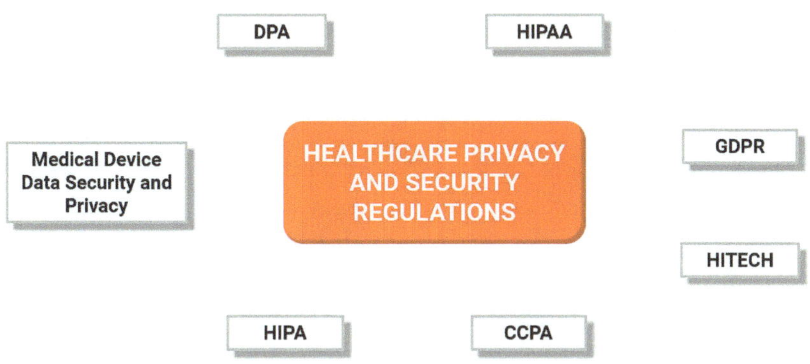

▼ **Figure 3.1:** Few Privacy Regulations

1. **Health Insurance Portability and Accountability Act (HIPAA):** HIPAA is a federal law in the United States that sets standards for the privacy, security, and confidentiality of individually identifiable health information. It applies to healthcare providers, health plans, and healthcare clearinghouses, as well as their business associates.

2. **Health Information Technology for Economic and Clinical Health (HITECH) Act:** The HITECH Act, enacted as part of the American Recovery and Reinvestment Act of 2009, focuses on the promotion of health information technology adoption and strengthening privacy and security protections for electronic health records (EHRs). It includes provisions for breach notification and increased penalties for non-compliance.

3. **General Data Protection Regulation (GDPR):** GDPR is a comprehensive data protection regulation in the European Union (EU) that applies to the processing of personal data, including healthcare information. It sets forth strict requirements for the lawful collection, use, and disclosure of personal data, along with robust privacy rights for individuals.

4. **California Consumer Privacy Act (CCPA):** The CCPA is a state-level privacy law in California, United States, that grants consumers certain rights regarding the collection, use, and sale of their personal information. It applies to many healthcare organizations that handle California residents' personal information.

5. **Health Information Protection Act (HIPA):** HIPA is a Canadian federal law that governs the protection of personal health information. It outlines the obligations of healthcare organizations, custodians, and service providers regarding the collection, use, and disclosure of personal health information.

6. **Data Protection Act 2018 (DPA):** The DPA is the primary data protection legislation in the United Kingdom. It includes provisions for protecting personal data, including health data, and implements the GDPR requirements within the UK context.

7. **Medical Device Data Security and Privacy:** Regulatory bodies, such as the U.S. Food and Drug Administration (FDA), issue guidelines and regulations specific to medical device data security and privacy. These regulations aim to ensure that medical devices, including those connected to networks or the Internet of Things (IoT), maintain appropriate safeguards to protect patient information.

It is important for healthcare organizations to understand and comply with these regulations to protect patient privacy and ensure the security of health information. Compliance with these regulations involves implementing appropriate administrative, technical, and physical safeguards, conducting risk assessments, providing employee training, and implementing data breach response protocols. Failure to comply with healthcare privacy and security regulations can result in significant penalties, reputational damage, and legal consequences.

Overview of Healthcare Privacy Laws (HIPAA, HITECH Act)

Healthcare privacy and security regulations are designed to protect the confidentiality, integrity, and availability of patients' health information. These regulations ensure that healthcare organizations handle personal health information responsibly and maintain appropriate safeguards to prevent unauthorized access, use, or disclosure. Here are further explanations of key healthcare privacy and security regulations:

1. **Health Insurance Portability and Accountability Act (HIPAA):**

   - HIPAA's Privacy Rule: The Privacy Rule establishes standards for the use and disclosure of protected health information (PHI). It grants individuals certain rights over their health information, including the right to access, amend, and request restrictions on the use of their PHI.

   - HIPAA's Security Rule: The Security Rule sets standards for protecting ePHI that is stored, transmitted, or processed electronically. It requires covered entities and business associates to implement safeguards to ensure the confidentiality, integrity, and availability of ePHI.

   - HIPAA's Breach Notification Rule: The Breach Notification Rule requires covered entities to notify affected individuals, HHS, and, in some cases, the media about breaches of unsecured PHI.

2. **Health Information Technology for Economic and Clinical Health (HITECH) Act:**

   - The HITECH Act promotes the adoption and meaningful use of electronic health records (EHRs) and strengthens the privacy and security protections for EHRs and ePHI.

   - It expanded the scope of HIPAA's Privacy and Security Rules to include business associates, such as vendors and subcontractors, who handle PHI on behalf of covered entities.

   - The HITECH Act introduced increased penalties for non-compliance with HIPAA, aligning penalties with the severity of the violation.

3. **General Data Protection Regulation (GDPR):**

   - The GDPR is a comprehensive data protection regulation applicable to organizations that handle the personal data of individuals in the European Union (EU).

   - It applies to healthcare organizations that collect, process, or store personal health information of EU residents.

   - The GDPR establishes strict requirements for lawful processing of personal data, including health data, and grants individuals enhanced privacy rights, such as the right to erasure and the right to data portability.

4. **California Consumer Privacy Act (CCPA):**

   - The CCPA is a state-level privacy law in California, United States, that grants consumers certain rights regarding the collection, use, and sale of their personal information.

   - It applies to many healthcare organizations that handle personal information of California residents, including PHI.

5. **Medical Device Data Security and Privacy:**

   - Regulatory bodies, such as the U.S. Food and Drug Administration (FDA), issue guidelines and regulations specific to medical device data security and privacy.

   - These regulations aim to ensure that medical devices, including those connected to networks or the Internet of Things (IoT), maintain appropriate safeguards to protect patient information.

Compliance with these regulations requires healthcare organizations to implement privacy and security measures, conduct risk assessments, train employees, maintain documentation, and respond appropriately to breaches or privacy incidents. Non-compliance can lead to significant penalties, reputational damage, and legal consequences.

Ensuring Patient Confidentiality and Data Security

Ensuring patient confidentiality and data security is of utmost importance in healthcare to maintain trust, protect sensitive information, and comply with privacy regulations. Here are key considerations for healthcare organizations to achieve this:

1. **Access Controls:** Implement strict access controls to ensure that patient information is only accessible to authorized individuals. This includes using unique user IDs, strong passwords, and two-factor authentication. Limit access to the minimum necessary information required for individual's job responsibilities.

2. **Data Encryption:** Encrypt sensitive patient data, both at rest and in transit, to protect it from unauthorized access. Use encryption technologies such

as Secure Sockets Layer (SSL) or Transport Layer Security (TLS) for data transmission and encryption protocols for data storage.

3. **Secure Data Storage:** Store patient data securely, whether in electronic health records (EHR) systems, databases, or physical files. Implement measures such as firewalls, intrusion detection systems, and regular security updates to protect against unauthorized access or breaches.

4. **Training and Awareness:** Provide comprehensive training and education to employees on patient confidentiality, data security, and privacy policies. Ensure that staff members understand the importance of protecting patient information and the potential consequences of mishandling or unauthorized disclosure.

5. **Privacy Policies and Consent:** Develop clear and comprehensive privacy policies that outline how patient information is collected, used, and disclosed. Obtain informed consent from patients for the collection and sharing of their data, ensuring transparency and compliance with privacy regulations.

6. **Vendor and Third-Party Management:** Establish robust contracts and agreements with vendors and third-party service providers to ensure they adhere to privacy and security standards. Regularly assess and monitor their compliance with data protection requirements.

7. **Data Breach Response Plan:** Develop a data breach response plan that outlines the steps to be taken in the event of a security incident or breach. This includes promptly notifying affected individuals, regulatory authorities, and implementing measures to mitigate the impact of the breach.

8. **Auditing and Monitoring:** Conduct regular audits and monitoring of systems, processes, and employee activities to detect any unauthorized access, data breaches, or policy violations. Implement logging mechanisms and utilize security information and event management (SIEM) tools to monitor for suspicious activities.

9. **Physical Security Measures:** Implement physical security measures, such as restricted access to sensitive areas, secure storage of physical files, and surveillance systems to prevent unauthorized access to patient information.

10. **Continuous Improvement and Risk Assessment:** Regularly assess risks to patient confidentiality and data security, taking into account evolving technologies, new threats, and regulatory changes. Continuously improve

security measures by addressing identified vulnerabilities, conducting risk assessments, and implementing appropriate controls.

By implementing these measures, healthcare organizations can prioritize patient confidentiality and data security, protect sensitive information, and maintain compliance with privacy regulations. This fosters trust among patients and ensures that their personal health information is handled responsibly and securely.

Implementing Electronic Health Records (EHR) and Safeguarding Patient Information

Implementing electronic health records (EHR) brings numerous benefits to healthcare organizations, including improved efficiency, accessibility, and coordination of patient information. However, safeguarding patient information within EHR systems is crucial to maintain data privacy and security. Here are key considerations for implementing EHR and safeguarding patient information:

1. **Access Controls:** Implement robust access controls within the EHR system to ensure that only authorized individuals can access patient information. This includes user authentication, role-based access control, and audit trails to monitor access activities.

2. **Encryption:** Encrypt patient data both at rest and in transit to protect it from unauthorized access. Utilize encryption technologies, such as SSL/TLS for data transmission and encryption protocols for data storage within the EHR system.

3. **Data Segmentation:** Implement data segmentation techniques to ensure that patient information is only accessible to authorized personnel based on their role and need-to-know basis. This prevents unnecessary exposure of sensitive information.

4. **User Training and Awareness:** Provide comprehensive training to users of the EHR system, including healthcare professionals and staff, on the importance of data privacy and security. Educate them about the proper handling, access, and sharing of patient information to mitigate risks.

5. **Audit and Monitoring:** Implement auditing and monitoring mechanisms within the EHR system to track and monitor user activities, access logs, and system logs. Regularly review audit logs to detect any unauthorized access or suspicious activities.

6. **Data Backup and Disaster Recovery:** Establish robust data backup and disaster recovery processes to ensure the availability and integrity of patient information. Regularly backup EHR data and test the restoration process to minimize data loss in the event of a system failure or disaster.

7. **Secure Authentication:** Implement strong authentication mechanisms, such as multi-factor authentication, to verify the identity of users accessing the EHR system. This helps prevent unauthorized access and potential breaches.

8. **Data Minimization:** Adopt a data minimization approach by collecting and storing only the necessary patient information within the EHR system. Avoid storing excessive or unnecessary data that could increase the risk of unauthorized access or data breaches.

9. **Vendor Security Assessment:** Assess the security measures implemented by EHR vendors before selecting a system. Ensure that the vendor follows industry best practices and complies with relevant security standards to safeguard patient information.

10. **Regular Risk Assessments:** Conduct regular risk assessments to identify vulnerabilities and potential threats to the security of patient information within the EHR system. Mitigate risks by implementing appropriate controls and continuously monitoring the system for any emerging security issues.

By implementing these considerations, healthcare organizations can effectively implement EHR systems while safeguarding patient information. This ensures data privacy, confidentiality, and security, promoting trust between healthcare providers and patients while complying with privacy regulations.

Responding to Data Breaches and Maintaining Breach Notification Protocols

Responding to data breaches and maintaining breach notification protocols are critical aspects of safeguarding patient information and complying with privacy regulations. Here are key considerations for responding to data breaches and maintaining breach notification protocols in healthcare:

1. **Establish a Data Breach Response Team:** Form a dedicated team that includes representatives from IT, legal, compliance, and communications departments to handle data breaches. This team will be responsible for coordinating breach response efforts.

2. **Contain and Mitigate the Breach:** Act swiftly to contain the breach and mitigate its impact. Identify the cause and extent of the breach, assess potential risks to patient information, and take immediate steps to prevent further unauthorized access or disclosure.

3. **Document the Incident:** Maintain a thorough record of the breach incident, including the date, time, and nature of the breach, as well as actions taken to respond and mitigate the breach. Document any evidence, logs, or other relevant information related to the breach.

4. **Assess Potential Harm:** Conduct a risk assessment to determine the potential harm or impact on affected individuals. Assess the types of information exposed, the likelihood of harm, and any mitigating factors to guide subsequent actions.

5. **Notify Affected Individuals:** Comply with breach notification requirements by promptly notifying affected individuals whose personal information has been compromised. Provide clear and concise information about the breach, potential risks, and steps individuals can take to protect themselves.

6. **Notify Relevant Authorities:** Comply with regulatory requirements by reporting the breach to the appropriate regulatory authorities. Understand the specific notification requirements of relevant regulatory bodies and ensure compliance with their timelines and procedures.

7. **Implement Corrective Actions:** Take appropriate corrective actions to address the breach and prevent similar incidents in the future. This may involve strengthening security controls, enhancing employee training, conducting internal investigations, or revising policies and procedures.

8. **Communicate with Stakeholders:** Establish effective communication channels to keep stakeholders informed about the breach, response efforts, and mitigation measures. This includes internal communication with staff, communication with affected individuals, and, if necessary, external communication with the media or public.

9. **Collaborate with Law Enforcement and Forensic Experts:** Engage with law enforcement agencies and forensic experts to investigate the breach, gather evidence, and identify the perpetrators. Cooperate fully with authorities to ensure a thorough investigation.

10. **Learn from the Incident:** Conduct a post-incident analysis to identify lessons learned from the breach. Evaluate response efforts, identify areas for

improvement, and implement changes to policies, procedures, and security controls to enhance data breach prevention and response capabilities.

By following these considerations, healthcare organizations can effectively respond to data breaches, minimize the impact on affected individuals, and maintain compliance with breach notification protocols. Prompt and thorough response to breaches helps preserve trust and confidentiality, demonstrating a commitment to protecting patient information.

Quality and Patient Safety Standards

Quality and patient safety standards are guidelines and principles established to ensure that healthcare organizations deliver safe, effective, and high-quality care to patients. These standards aim to minimize medical errors, prevent harm, and improve patient outcomes. Here are some key aspects of quality and patient safety standards:

1. **Evidence-Based Practice:** Quality and patient safety standards are grounded in evidence-based practice, which means healthcare decisions and practices are informed by the best available scientific evidence. Healthcare organizations are encouraged to adopt evidence-based guidelines and protocols to ensure that care is based on the most current knowledge and research.

2. **Clinical Guidelines:** Clinical guidelines are evidence-based recommendations for healthcare providers to follow in the diagnosis, treatment, and management of various medical conditions. These guidelines help standardize care, promote best practices, and improve patient outcomes by ensuring that healthcare professionals are delivering care based on the latest research and expert consensus.

3. **Patient-Centered Care:** Quality and patient safety standards emphasize the importance of patient-centered care, which involves actively involving patients in their healthcare decisions, respecting their preferences and values, and promoting open communication and shared decision-making. Patient-centered care focuses on the individual needs, goals, and preferences of patients, enhancing their experience and satisfaction.

4. **Performance Measurement and Reporting:** Quality and patient safety standards often require healthcare organizations to measure and report their performance using specific metrics and indicators. These measures

may include patient outcomes (e.g., mortality rates, readmission rates), patient satisfaction surveys, adherence to clinical protocols, and other quality-related indicators. Performance measurement helps identify areas for improvement and allows for benchmarking and comparisons with peers.

5. **Patient Safety Culture:** Quality and patient safety standards emphasize the importance of fostering a culture of safety within healthcare organizations. This involves creating an environment where all staff members feel comfortable reporting errors or near misses, promoting open and transparent communication, encouraging a blame-free approach to errors, and implementing systems for learning from mistakes and preventing future occurrences.

6. **Risk Management and Incident Reporting:** Healthcare organizations are required to have robust risk management systems and processes in place to identify and mitigate potential risks to patient safety. This includes encouraging staff to report incidents and near misses, conducting thorough investigations into adverse events, implementing corrective actions, and using the information learned to improve systems and prevent future errors.

7. **Regulatory and Accreditation Standards:** Regulatory bodies and accrediting organizations play a crucial role in setting quality and patient safety standards. They develop guidelines, standards, and regulations that healthcare organizations must adhere to in order to maintain compliance. Examples include The Joint Commission (TJC) in the United States and the Care Quality Commission (CQC) in the United Kingdom.

8. **Continuous Quality Improvement:** Quality and patient safety standards emphasize the importance of continuous quality improvement. Healthcare organizations are encouraged to regularly assess their performance, identify areas for improvement, implement changes, and monitor the impact of those changes. This iterative process of continuous improvement helps enhance care delivery, patient outcomes, and safety over time.

By adhering to quality and patient safety standards, healthcare organizations can ensure that they provide safe, effective, and patient-centered care. These standards help drive improvements in clinical outcomes, enhance patient satisfaction, and reduce the risk of adverse events, ultimately leading to better overall healthcare quality and safety.

Introduction to Quality Improvement Initiatives in Healthcare

Quality improvement initiatives in healthcare are systematic efforts aimed at enhancing the delivery of care, improving patient outcomes, and optimizing healthcare processes. These initiatives focus on identifying areas for improvement, implementing evidence-based practices, and measuring and monitoring performance to achieve better results. Here are key aspects of quality improvement initiatives (Table 4.1):

▼ **Table 4.1:** Key Quality Standards and Initiatives

Quality Standard/Initiative	Description
Accreditation Standards (e.g., Joint Commission)	Set of performance standards that healthcare organizations must meet to receive accreditation.
National Patient Safety Goals	Prioritized areas of focus for patient safety improvement established by organizations like the Joint Commission.
Healthcare-associated Infection (HAI) Measures	Metrics used to monitor and reduce the occurrence of healthcare-associated infections, such as Central Line-Associated Bloodstream Infections (CLABSIs) and Catheter-Associated Urinary Tract Infections (CAUTIs).
Core Measures	Set of evidence-based quality measures for common conditions and procedures, including measures related to heart attacks, pneumonia, surgical care, and more.

1. **Continuous Improvement:** Quality improvement initiatives embrace the concept of continuous improvement, recognizing that healthcare is an evolving field and that there is always room for improvement. It involves an ongoing cycle of assessment, planning, implementation, and evaluation to drive positive change.

2. **Data-Driven Approach:** Quality improvement initiatives rely on data collection, analysis, and measurement to identify gaps, assess performance, and track progress. Quality metrics, indicators, and

performance measures are used to monitor outcomes, identify trends, and inform decision-making.

3. **Evidence-Based Practice:** Quality improvement initiatives emphasize the use of evidence-based practices. They leverage scientific research, clinical guidelines, and best practices to inform the development and implementation of interventions and processes aimed at improving patient care and outcomes.

4. **Patient-Centeredness:** Quality improvement initiatives prioritize patient-centered care. They strive to engage patients and their families in decision-making, address individual needs and preferences, and promote patient satisfaction and experience as essential components of high-quality care.

5. **Interdisciplinary Collaboration:** Quality improvement initiatives involve collaboration among multidisciplinary healthcare teams. They bring together healthcare professionals from various specialties and disciplines to collectively work towards improving processes, communication, and coordination of care.

6. **Quality Measurement and Reporting:** Quality improvement initiatives involve the measurement and reporting of performance indicators and quality metrics. This includes tracking outcomes, adherence to guidelines, patient satisfaction, and other relevant measures to assess the effectiveness of interventions and drive improvements.

7. **Plan-Do-Study-Act (PDSA) Cycle:** The Plan-Do-Study-Act (PDSA) cycle is a widely used quality improvement methodology. It involves developing a plan, implementing changes, studying the outcomes through data analysis, and acting upon the findings to refine and sustain improvements.

8. **Benchmarking and Collaboration:** Quality improvement initiatives often involve benchmarking, which is the process of comparing performance against recognized standards or peers. Sharing best practices and collaborating with other organizations can help identify innovative approaches and drive improvement across the healthcare system.

9. **Leadership and Culture:** Effective quality improvement initiatives require leadership commitment and a culture that values continuous learning, transparency, and accountability. Leadership support fosters a culture of quality and promotes engagement among staff members to drive change and sustain improvements.

By embracing quality improvement initiatives, healthcare organizations can enhance patient outcomes, optimize processes, and deliver care that is evidence-based, patient-centered, and continuously improving. These initiatives contribute to the overall goal of providing high-quality healthcare services to individuals and communities.

Compliance with Quality Standards

Compliance with quality standards is crucial for healthcare organizations to ensure that they meet established benchmarks and deliver high-quality care. Adhering to quality standards helps organizations improve patient outcomes, enhance patient safety, and provide consistent and effective care. Here are key aspects of compliance with quality standards:

1. **Regulatory and Accreditation Standards:** Healthcare organizations must comply with regulatory requirements and accreditation standards set by government agencies and accrediting bodies. These standards may include specific guidelines for clinical practices, patient safety protocols, infection control measures, and data reporting.

2. **National Quality Initiatives:** Many countries have national quality initiatives aimed at improving healthcare quality and patient outcomes. Healthcare organizations should align their practices with these initiatives and follow the guidelines and recommendations provided.

3. **Quality Metrics and Indicators:** Compliance with quality standards involves measuring and monitoring performance using quality metrics and indicators. These metrics may include patient outcomes, patient satisfaction, adherence to clinical guidelines, infection rates, and other quality-related measures. Regular tracking and reporting of these metrics help identify areas for improvement and demonstrate compliance with quality standards.

4. **Quality Improvement Programs:** Implementing quality improvement programs is essential for compliance with quality standards. These programs involve assessing current practices, identifying gaps, implementing evidence-based interventions, and continuously monitoring outcomes to drive improvement. Compliance with quality standards requires active participation in quality improvement initiatives.

5. **Clinical Documentation and Record-Keeping:** Accurate and complete clinical documentation is crucial for quality compliance. Healthcare organizations must maintain comprehensive and up-to-date patient records, including diagnoses, treatment plans, medication records, and other relevant information. Proper documentation ensures continuity of care, facilitates communication among healthcare providers, and supports accurate reporting of quality indicators.

6. **Staff Training and Education:** Compliance with quality standards necessitates ongoing training and education for healthcare professionals. Staff members should receive training on best practices, quality improvement methodologies, patient safety protocols, and compliance with regulatory and accreditation requirements. Education programs help ensure that all staff members are knowledgeable about quality standards and contribute to their implementation.

7. **Internal Audits and Assessments:** Conducting internal audits and assessments is vital for ensuring compliance with quality standards. Regular self-assessment and evaluation of processes, policies, and outcomes help identify areas of non-compliance and areas for improvement. Internal audits provide an opportunity to address gaps, implement corrective actions, and monitor progress towards meeting quality standards.

8. **External Review and Accreditation Surveys:** Healthcare organizations undergo external reviews and accreditation surveys to assess compliance with quality standards. Accrediting bodies and regulatory agencies conduct inspections and assessments to evaluate adherence to quality guidelines. Compliance with these external reviews ensures that the organization meets recognized standards and demonstrates a commitment to quality care.

9. **Quality Reporting and Transparency:** Compliance with quality standards involves transparently reporting quality data and outcomes to stakeholders, including patients, regulatory bodies, accrediting agencies, and the public. This transparency promotes accountability, fosters trust, and allows for comparisons against peers or benchmarks.

By actively complying with quality standards, healthcare organizations can provide consistent, safe, and effective care to patients. Compliance supports the delivery of high-quality services, improves patient satisfaction, and contributes to better health outcomes for individuals and communities.

Patient Safety Regulations and Strategies for Error Prevention

Patient safety regulations and strategies for error prevention are essential components of healthcare systems to ensure the well-being and safety of patients. These regulations and strategies aim to minimize the occurrence of medical errors, prevent harm, and promote a culture of safety within healthcare organizations. Here are key aspects of patient safety regulations and strategies for error prevention (Table 4.2):

▼ **Table 4.2:** Quality Improvement Tools and Methodologies

Tool/Methodology	Description
Plan-Do-Study-Act (PDSA) Cycle	A structured approach for testing and implementing changes in healthcare processes to improve quality and safety.
Root Cause Analysis (RCA)	A systematic method for identifying the underlying causes of adverse events or near misses and developing corrective actions to prevent recurrence.
Failure Mode and Effects Analysis (FMEA)	A proactive approach for identifying potential failures and their impact on patient safety, analyzing their causes, and implementing preventive measures.
Lean Six Sigma	A methodology combining Lean principles (reducing waste) and Six Sigma (reducing process variation) to enhance quality, efficiency, and patient safety.

1. **Regulatory Frameworks:** Regulatory bodies, such as government agencies or healthcare commissions, establish patient safety regulations and guidelines to promote safe practices and minimize risks. These regulations may include requirements for infection control, medication safety, surgical procedures, documentation standards, and reporting of adverse events.

2. **Medication Safety:** Strategies for medication safety focus on reducing medication errors, such as prescribing errors, administration errors, or medication reconciliation discrepancies. These strategies involve implementing electronic prescribing systems, barcode scanning for medication

administration, standardized medication labeling, and clear communication among healthcare providers.

3. **Healthcare-Associated Infections (HAIs) Prevention:** HAIs are a significant concern in healthcare settings. Strategies for preventing HAIs include strict adherence to hand hygiene protocols, proper sterilization and disinfection of medical equipment, implementation of infection control protocols, and surveillance systems to detect and respond to potential outbreaks.

4. **Surgical Safety:** Surgical safety strategies aim to minimize surgical errors and prevent adverse events during surgical procedures. This involves implementing surgical checklists, proper preoperative verification processes, site marking protocols, and time-outs to verify patient and procedure details before surgery.

5. **Communication and Teamwork:** Effective communication and teamwork are crucial for error prevention. Strategies focus on enhancing communication among healthcare professionals, promoting a culture of open dialogue, and encouraging the reporting of near misses and adverse events. Implementing standardized communication protocols, such as the use of SBAR (Situation, Background, Assessment, Recommendation), helps improve clarity and prevent miscommunication.

6. **Error Reporting and Learning Systems:** Establishing error reporting systems and learning from mistakes are vital for error prevention. Healthcare organizations should encourage staff members to report errors and near misses without fear of reprisal. These reported incidents are analyzed through root cause analysis and contribute to organizational learning and system improvements to prevent similar errors in the future.

7. **Patient Engagement:** Engaging patients in their care is an important strategy for error prevention. Encouraging patients to actively participate in their treatment decisions, providing clear and understandable information, and promoting shared decision-making can help identify and prevent potential errors or misunderstandings.

8. **Staff Education and Training:** Ongoing education and training for healthcare professionals are essential for error prevention. This includes training on patient safety principles, error recognition and reporting, proper use of medical devices, infection control practices, and other specific strategies to minimize risks and promote safe practices.

9. **Root Cause Analysis and Process Improvement:** Conducting root cause analysis when errors or adverse events occur helps identify underlying causes and contributing factors. These analyses guide process improvements and the implementation of preventive measures to mitigate future risks and prevent similar errors.

10. **Technology and Automation:** Utilizing technology and automation can play a significant role in error prevention. This includes electronic health records (EHRs) for accurate and up-to-date patient information, computerized physician order entry (CPOE) systems to reduce prescribing errors, bar-coding systems for medication administration, and decision support tools to provide real-time alerts and guidance to healthcare providers.

By implementing patient safety regulations and strategies for error prevention, healthcare organizations can create safer environments, reduce the occurrence of medical errors, and improve patient outcomes. These initiatives foster a culture of safety and continuous improvement, ensuring the well-being of patients and the delivery of high-quality care.

Monitoring Adverse Events and Implementing Root Cause Analysis

Monitoring adverse events and implementing root cause analysis are critical components of patient safety initiatives in healthcare. These practices help healthcare organizations identify and address the underlying causes of adverse events, prevent their recurrence, and improve patient safety. Here are key aspects of monitoring adverse events and implementing root cause analysis:

1. **Adverse Event Monitoring:**

   - Establish a system for reporting adverse events and near misses. Encourage healthcare professionals to report incidents without fear of reprisal.

   - Utilize incident reporting tools or electronic systems to capture and track adverse events.

   - Regularly analyze reported events to identify patterns, trends, and potential areas for improvement.

   - Monitor adverse events based on severity, type (e.g., medication errors, falls, infections), and location within the healthcare organization.

- Consider external sources of data, such as patient feedback, complaints, and satisfaction surveys, to supplement internal monitoring efforts.

2. **Root Cause Analysis (RCA):**

   - Conduct root cause analysis for significant adverse events or near misses to understand the underlying causes and contributing factors.

   - Form a multidisciplinary team with expertise in relevant areas, including clinicians, administrators, quality improvement specialists, and patient safety experts.

   - Utilize structured methodologies (e.g., Fish-bone diagram, 5 Whys, Cause and Effect Analysis) to systematically identify root causes.

   - Gather and analyze data, including medical records, incident reports, witness accounts, and relevant policies and procedures.

   - Identify both immediate and underlying causes, including system failures, communication breakdowns, human factors, and organizational issues.

   - Prioritize root causes based on their potential to prevent similar adverse events and focus improvement efforts accordingly.

3. **Preventive Measures:**

- Develop and implement action plans to address identified root causes and prevent recurrence of adverse events.

- Engage stakeholders, including frontline staff, in the design and implementation of preventive measures.

- Establish strategies and interventions to address system-level issues, improve communication and teamwork, enhance processes, and promote a culture of safety.

- Monitor the effectiveness of preventive measures and adjust interventions as needed.

- Share lessons learned and best practices with the organization to enhance learning and improve patient safety.

4. **Continuous Learning and Improvement:**

- Use the findings from adverse event monitoring and root cause analysis to drive organizational learning and continuous improvement.

- Establish mechanisms for sharing RCA outcomes and recommendations across departments and units.

- Incorporate the lessons learned into training programs, policies, and procedures.

- Regularly review and update protocols and guidelines based on identified root causes and best practices.

- Foster a culture that encourages reporting and learning from adverse events, creating an environment of transparency, accountability, and continuous improvement.

Monitoring adverse events and implementing root cause analysis are essential in identifying and addressing the underlying causes of patient safety incidents. These practices enable healthcare organizations to develop targeted interventions, enhance processes, and improve patient outcomes by preventing the recurrence of similar adverse events.

Chapter 05

Billing and Coding Compliance

Billing and coding compliance refers to the adherence to regulations, guidelines, and ethical standards in accurately documenting and reporting healthcare services for reimbursement purposes. It involves the proper assignment of diagnostic and procedural codes, ensuring that the documentation supports the services billed, and following the applicable billing rules and regulations. Compliance with billing and coding standards is crucial for healthcare organizations to receive appropriate reimbursement, prevent fraud and abuse, and maintain legal and regulatory compliance. Here are key aspects of billing and coding compliance:

1. **Coding Accuracy:** Accurate coding is essential for proper reimbursement and effective communication of patient diagnoses and procedures. It involves assigning the correct codes based on the documentation provided by healthcare providers. Coding accuracy ensures that the services rendered are adequately described and supported by clinical documentation.

2. **Documentation Requirements:** Accurate and comprehensive documentation is the foundation of billing and coding compliance. Healthcare providers must document all relevant patient encounters, including diagnoses, procedures, treatments, and any other pertinent information. Documentation should be clear, complete, and reflect the medical necessity of the services provided.

3. **Coding Guidelines and Conventions:** Billing and coding compliance requires adherence to coding guidelines and conventions specific to each coding system. This includes understanding and applying the Official Coding Guidelines, CPT guidelines, HCPCS guidelines, and any other applicable coding rules. Adhering to these guidelines ensures consistent and standardized coding practices.

4. **Regulatory and Payer Requirements:** Compliance with billing and coding regulations is essential to meet the requirements set by regulatory bodies and payers. This includes adherence to regulations such as the Centers for Medicare and Medicaid Services (CMS) guidelines, local coverage determinations (LCDs), and payer-specific policies. Understanding and following these requirements minimize the risk of improper billing and potential audit findings.

5. **Medical Necessity:** Billing and coding compliance requires the documentation and coding of services that meet the criteria of medical necessity. Medical necessity refers to the reasonable and necessary services that are appropriate for the patient's condition and supported by clinical documentation. Ensuring that services meet medical necessity criteria helps prevent over billing and potential audits.

6. **Claims Submission and Reimbursement:** Compliance with billing and coding regulations includes accurately submitting claims and seeking reimbursement for services provided. This involves timely and accurate claim submission, appropriate use of modifiers, inclusion of required documentation, and adherence to payer-specific billing rules. Compliance with reimbursement guidelines ensures proper payment for services rendered.

7. **Auditing and Monitoring:** Healthcare organizations must implement internal auditing and monitoring processes to ensure ongoing compliance with billing and coding standards. Regular audits help identify potential coding errors, documentation deficiencies, and areas for improvement. Monitoring coding accuracy and compliance helps address any identified issues promptly and prevent future compliance problems.

8. **Ethical and Legal Considerations:** Billing and coding compliance also involves ethical and legal considerations. Healthcare professionals must adhere to professional codes of conduct, avoid fraudulent practices, and maintain patient confidentiality. Compliance with privacy and security regulations, such as HIPAA, is critical in safeguarding patient information.

By prioritizing billing and coding compliance, healthcare organizations can mitigate risks, maintain financial integrity, and ensure accurate reimbursement for the services provided. Adhering to coding guidelines, documenting services appropriately, and staying updated on regulatory changes contribute to ethical billing practices and overall healthcare compliance.

Overview of Billing and Coding Regulations (CMS Guidelines, CPT Codes, ICD-10)

Billing and coding regulations provide guidelines and standards for accurately documenting and reporting healthcare services for reimbursement purposes. These regulations ensure consistency, accuracy, and compliance in the billing and coding process. Here's an overview of key regulations in the field (Table 5.1):

▼ **Table 5.1:** Common Billing and Coding Regulations

Regulation	Description
CMS Guidelines	Centers for Medicare and Medicaid Services (CMS) guidelines for billing and coding practices.
CPT Codes	Current Procedural Terminology (CPT) codes used for reporting medical procedures and services.
ICD-10 Codes	International Classification of Diseases, 10th Revision (ICD-10) codes for diagnosis coding.
E/M Documentation Guidelines	Evaluation and Management (E/M) documentation guidelines for accurately reporting patient visits.

1. **Centers for Medicare and Medicaid Services (CMS) Guidelines:** CMS is a federal agency that administers the Medicare and Medicaid programs. It provides guidelines and regulations for billing and coding practices in these programs. CMS guidelines include:

   - Medicare Claims Processing Manual: Outlines the rules and procedures for submitting claims, including documentation requirements, coding guidelines, and reimbursement methodologies.

   - National Coverage Determinations (NCDs): Specify the conditions under which Medicare provides coverage for certain services or procedures.

   - Local Coverage Determinations (LCDs): Developed by Medicare Administrative Contractors (MACs) and provide specific coverage guidelines for local regions.

2. **Current Procedural Terminology (CPT) Codes:** CPT codes are a set of codes developed and maintained by the American Medical Association (AMA). They describe medical procedures and services performed by healthcare professionals. CPT codes are widely used in the United States for

billing and reimbursement purposes. Each CPT code represents a specific procedure or service and is associated with a corresponding description and reimbursement value.

3. **International Classification of Diseases, Tenth Revision (ICD-10):** The ICD-10 is a diagnostic coding system used globally to classify diseases, injuries, and other health conditions. It provides a standardized way of documenting patient diagnoses. ICD-10 codes are alphanumeric and include details about the diagnosis, its severity, and any relevant factors. Accurate ICD-10 coding is crucial for ensuring appropriate reimbursement and supporting medical necessity.

4. **HIPAA Transaction and Code Set Rules:** The Health Insurance Portability and Accountability Act (HIPAA) includes rules related to the electronic exchange of healthcare transactions, including billing and coding. The HIPAA Transaction and Code Set Rules set standards for electronic claims submission, code sets (such as CPT and ICD-10), and other transactional requirements.

5. **National Correct Coding Initiative (NCCI):** NCCI is a CMS program that promotes correct coding practices and prevents improper payment due to coding errors. NCCI edits identify code combinations that should not be reported together unless specific circumstances exist. Adhering to NCCI guidelines helps prevent billing and coding errors and ensures appropriate reimbursement

6. **Local Coverage Determinations (LCDs):** LCDs are developed by MACs, which are contracted by CMS to process Medicare claims. LCDs provide region-specific guidelines for coverage and reimbursement of services. They outline medical necessity criteria, coding requirements, and documentation expectations for specific procedures or conditions.

7. **Other Payer-Specific Guidelines:** Different insurance payers, such as commercial insurers and Medicaid programs, may have their own specific billing and coding guidelines. These guidelines may include additional requirements, coverage policies, and documentation standards that healthcare providers must follow when submitting claims to those payers.

Compliance with billing and coding regulations is crucial for healthcare organizations to ensure accurate reimbursement, prevent fraud and abuse, and maintain legal and regulatory compliance. Healthcare professionals and organizations should stay updated on the latest guidelines and regulations to ensure compliance with billing and coding practices and optimize reimbursement for services provided.

Ensuring Accurate Coding and Documentation Practices

Ensuring accurate coding and documentation practices is essential for healthcare organizations to support proper reimbursement, facilitate effective communication, and maintain compliance with billing and coding regulations. Here are key strategies for ensuring accuracy in coding and documentation:

1. **Education and Training:** Provide comprehensive education and training to healthcare professionals involved in coding and documentation. Ensure they have a solid understanding of coding guidelines, documentation requirements, and relevant regulations. Ongoing training keeps staff up to date with changes in coding systems and best practices.

2. **Clear Documentation Guidelines:** Establish clear and concise documentation guidelines that outline the required elements for accurate coding. Ensure healthcare professionals understand the importance of complete, detailed, and specific documentation to support the services provided.

3. **Clinical Documentation Improvement (CDI) Programs:** Implement CDI programs to enhance documentation practices. CDI specialists work closely with healthcare providers to ensure accurate and comprehensive documentation that captures the complexity and specificity of patient conditions and treatments.

4. **Collaboration between Coding and Clinical Staff:** Foster collaboration between coding professionals and clinical staff to ensure accurate coding. Encourage open communication and provide a platform for coders to seek clarification or additional information from clinicians when necessary.

5. **Regular Audits and Feedback:** Conduct regular internal audits of coding and documentation practices to identify areas for improvement and address any inaccuracies or deficiencies. Provide feedback to healthcare professionals regarding coding accuracy and documentation completeness, and offer guidance for improvement.

6. **Coding Compliance Reviews:** Perform coding compliance reviews to assess coding accuracy and compliance with regulatory requirements. These reviews help identify potential coding errors, documentation gaps, and areas of improvement. Address any identified issues through appropriate education, training, and corrective actions.

7. **Use of Coding Software and Tools:** Utilize coding software and tools that incorporate coding guidelines and alerts for potential errors or inconsistencies. These tools can help improve coding accuracy, automate code searches, and enhance documentation support.

8. **Regular Coding and Documentation Audits by External Entities:** Engage external entities, such as coding consultants or auditing firms, to perform periodic coding and documentation audits. These audits provide an unbiased assessment of coding accuracy and adherence to regulatory requirements, highlighting areas for improvement and ensuring compliance.

9. **Continuous Communication and Updates:** Stay informed about changes in coding guidelines, regulations, and payer requirements. Communicate updates to coding and clinical staff promptly to ensure accurate coding and documentation practices. Regularly review coding-related publications, attend educational seminars, and participate in professional coding associations to stay updated on industry changes.

10. **Compliance Monitoring and Corrective Actions:** Establish mechanisms to monitor compliance with coding and documentation practices. Implement corrective actions to address identified issues and ensure adherence to regulatory requirements. This may include additional training, process improvements, and ongoing monitoring to sustain accuracy over time.

By implementing these strategies, healthcare organizations can promote accurate coding and documentation practices, support appropriate reimbursement, reduce coding errors, and maintain compliance with billing and coding regulations. Accurate coding and documentation contribute to improved patient care, effective communication, and optimized financial outcomes.

Strategies for Preventing Fraud and Abuse (False Claims Act, Stark Law, Anti-Kickback Statute)

Preventing fraud and abuse is crucial in healthcare to protect patients, maintain the integrity of the healthcare system, and comply with legal and regulatory requirements. Here are key strategies for preventing fraud and abuse, focusing on three important laws (Table 5.2):

▼ **Table 5.2:** Fraud and Abuse Laws and Regulations

Law/Regulation	Description
False Claims Act	Federal law prohibiting the submission of false claims to government healthcare programs.
Stark Law	Prohibits physician self-referral for certain designated health services to prevent conflicts of interest.
Anti-Kickback Statute	Prohibits offering, receiving, or soliciting remuneration in exchange for referrals or healthcare services.
Exclusion Authorities	Laws allowing the government to exclude individuals or entities from participating in federal healthcare programs.

1. **False Claims Act (FCA):**

   - Implement an effective compliance program: Establish a comprehensive compliance program that includes policies, procedures, and training to prevent and detect fraud and abuse. The program should include mechanisms for reporting suspected violations and conducting internal investigations.

   - Ensure accurate billing and coding practices: Adhere to coding guidelines, document services accurately, and bill only for services actually provided and supported by appropriate documentation. Conduct regular audits to identify coding errors or improper billing practices.

   - Monitor and address compliance risks: Conduct risk assessments to identify potential areas of fraud and abuse. Regularly monitor billing patterns, billing errors, and outlier cases. Develop strategies to address identified risks and implement corrective actions.

2. **Stark Law (Physician Self-Referral Law):**

   - Prohibit physician self-referrals: Ensure compliance with the Stark Law's prohibition on physicians referring patients to entities in which they have a financial relationship, unless an exception applies. Implement internal controls to prevent self-referral and maintain documentation of any permissible arrangements.

   - Establish fair market value and commercial reasonableness: Ensure that financial relationships between physicians and entities are based on fair market value and are commercially reasonable. Conduct regular valuations and assessments of these relationships to ensure compliance.

- Monitor and manage compensation arrangements: Regularly review and assess physician compensation arrangements to ensure compliance with Stark Law requirements. Establish clear policies and documentation processes for compensation agreements with physicians.

3. **Anti-Kickback Statute:**

- Prohibit kickbacks and inducements: Avoid offering, soliciting, or accepting any remuneration intended to induce referrals or generate business. Establish policies and procedures to prevent illegal kickback arrangements and educate employees on the requirements and implications of the Anti-Kickback Statute.

- Develop compliant financial relationships: Ensure financial relationships, such as contracts or arrangements with referral sources, comply with safe harbors or other exceptions provided under the Anti-Kickback Statute. Document and maintain evidence of compliance with these exceptions.

- Conduct regular compliance audits: Perform periodic audits to monitor compliance with the Anti-Kickback Statute. Evaluate financial relationships, referral patterns, and remuneration arrangements to identify potential violations. Promptly address any identified issues and implement corrective actions.

Additional Strategies:

- Employee education and training: Train employees on fraud and abuse laws, their responsibilities, and the consequences of non-compliance. Provide regular updates and reminders to keep staff informed about relevant laws and regulations.

- Confidential reporting mechanisms: Establish confidential reporting mechanisms, such as hotlines or anonymous reporting channels, to encourage employees to report suspected fraud or abuse. Ensure non-retaliation policies protect employees who report concerns in good faith.

- Independent audits and external reviews: Engage external auditors or consultants to perform independent audits and reviews of compliance programs, billing practices, and financial relationships. External reviews provide objective assessments and identify areas for improvement.

- Collaboration with regulatory authorities: Establish collaborative relationships with regulatory authorities, such as the Office of Inspector General (OIG), and proactively engage in dialogue to seek guidance and clarification on compliance matters.

By implementing these strategies, healthcare organizations can promote a culture of compliance, prevent fraud and abuse, and protect their reputation and financial stability. Regular monitoring, ongoing education, and proactive compliance efforts are essential to ensure adherence to legal and regulatory requirements.

Conducting Internal Audits and Responding to External Audits

Internal audits and external audits play a crucial role in ensuring compliance with regulations, identifying areas of improvement, and mitigating risks related to fraud, abuse, and billing inaccuracies. Here are key considerations for conducting internal audits and responding to external audits (Figure 5.1):

Conducting Internal Audits:

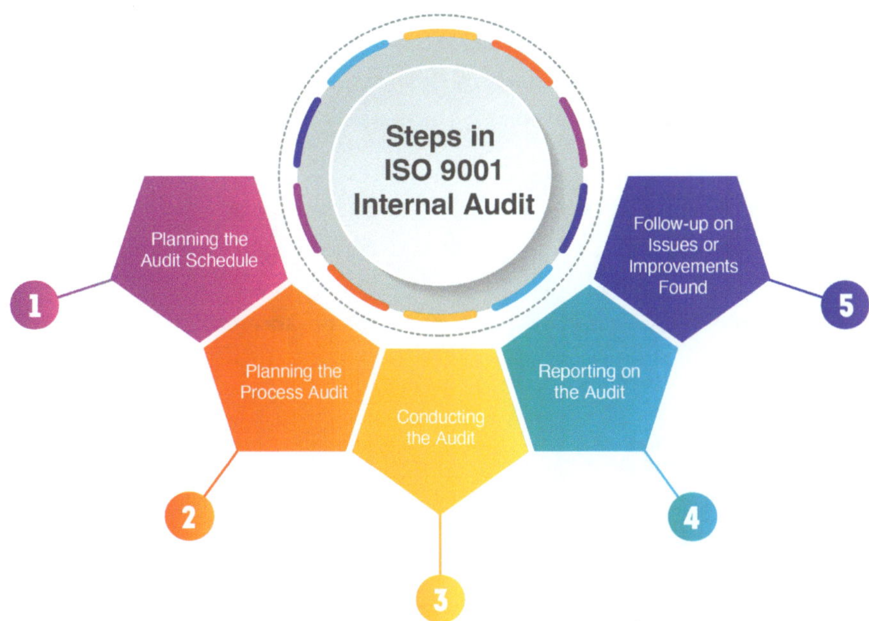

▼ **Figure 5.1:** Steps to Conduct Internal Audit

1. **Establish Audit Objectives:** Define the objectives of the internal audit, such as evaluating compliance with coding and billing regulations, identifying potential risks, or assessing the effectiveness of internal controls.

2. **Develop Audit Plan and Procedures:** Create a detailed audit plan that outlines the scope, methodology, and procedures to be followed during the audit. This may include reviewing medical records, claims data, billing practices, coding accuracy, and adherence to documentation requirements.

3. **Gather and Analyze Data:** Collect relevant data and documentation to support the audit objectives. This may involve reviewing medical records, financial records, billing data, coding documentation, and internal policies and procedures.

4. **Conduct Interviews and Discussions:** Interview key personnel involved in coding, billing, and compliance to gather additional information and insights. These discussions can help identify potential areas of non-compliance, system weaknesses, or process gaps.

5. **Assess Compliance with Regulations:** Evaluate compliance with relevant laws, regulations, and industry standards, including coding guidelines, documentation requirements, fraud and abuse laws, and billing regulations. Identify any instances of non-compliance or areas for improvement.

6. **Identify Risks and Control Weaknesses:** Identify potential risks related to fraud, abuse, or billing inaccuracies. Assess the effectiveness of internal controls in place and identify any weaknesses that may need to be addressed.

7. **Report Findings and Recommendations:** Prepare a comprehensive audit report that summarizes the findings, identifies areas of non-compliance, and provides recommendations for improvement. Share the report with relevant stakeholders, including management and compliance officers.

Responding to External Audits:

1. **Prepare for the Audit:** Review the audit notice or request and gather the necessary documentation and information in advance. Understand the scope and objectives of the external audit.

2. **Designate an Audit Coordinator:** Appoint an individual or team responsible for coordinating the audit process, serving as the main point of contact for the auditors, and facilitating the audit activities.

3. **Cooperate with Auditors:** Provide auditors with access to requested documents, information, and personnel. Cooperate fully during the audit process and address any questions or concerns raised by the auditors promptly and accurately.

4. **Maintain Communication:** Maintain open and transparent communication with the auditors throughout the audit process. Clarify any misunderstandings, provide additional information when requested, and address any concerns raised by the auditors.

5. **Address Findings and Recommendations:** Once the audit is completed, review the audit findings and recommendations provided by the external auditors. Develop and implement corrective actions to address any identified non-compliance or areas for improvement.

6. **Ensure Timely Responses:** Respond to the audit findings and recommendations within the specified timeframe. Provide a detailed response outlining the corrective actions taken or planned, along with a timeline for implementation.

7. **Monitor and Follow-Up:** Monitor the implementation of corrective actions and ensure ongoing compliance with the audit recommendations. Conduct internal follow-up audits to verify the effectiveness of the implemented changes.

By conducting thorough internal audits and effectively responding to external audits, healthcare organizations can identify compliance gaps, mitigate risks, improve processes, and ensure adherence to regulatory requirements. Internal and external audits provide opportunities for continuous improvement, support compliance efforts, and help safeguard the integrity of billing and coding practices.

Pharmaceutical and Medical Device Regulations

Pharmaceutical and medical device regulations are put in place to ensure the safety, efficacy, and quality of drugs and medical devices, protect public health, and provide a framework for their development, manufacturing, distribution, and marketing. Here's an overview of key aspects of pharmaceutical and medical device regulations:

Pharmaceutical Regulations:

1. **Food and Drug Administration (FDA):** In the United States, the FDA is the primary regulatory body responsible for overseeing pharmaceutical products. The FDA regulates the development, manufacturing, labeling, and marketing of drugs. It reviews and approves new drug applications, monitors drug safety, and enforces compliance with regulations.

2. **Drug Development Process:** Pharmaceutical regulations outline the requirements for the development and approval of drugs. This includes pre-clinical studies, clinical trials, and submission of data to support safety, efficacy, and quality. Regulations specify the criteria for clinical trial design, patient enrollment, and data collection.

3. **Good Manufacturing Practices (GMP):** GMP regulations ensure that pharmaceutical manufacturers follow standardized procedures and maintain quality control throughout the manufacturing process. GMP guidelines cover areas such as facilities, equipment, personnel, documentation, quality control testing, and product labeling.

4. **Labeling and Packaging:** Regulations govern the labeling and packaging of pharmaceutical products to ensure accurate and clear information for healthcare professionals and patients. Requirements include drug name, dosage form, strength, indications, contraindications, warnings, and storage instructions.

5. **Post-Marketing Surveillance:** Pharmaceutical regulations require ongoing post-marketing surveillance to monitor the safety and efficacy of drugs once they are on the market. Manufacturers are obligated to report adverse events, conduct post-marketing studies, and update product labeling based on new safety information.

Medical Device Regulations:

1. **FDA Regulation:** The FDA is responsible for regulating medical devices in the United States. The FDA classifies medical devices into different categories based on risk, and regulations vary depending on the classification. The FDA reviews and approves pre-market submissions, sets performance standards, and monitors device safety and quality.

2. **Device Classification:** Medical devices are categorized into classes (Class I, II, or III) based on risk and level of control necessary to ensure safety and efficacy. Class I devices have the lowest risk, while Class III devices have the highest risk and undergo the most rigorous regulatory scrutiny.

3. **Quality System Regulations (QSR):** QSR outlines the requirements for the design, manufacturing, packaging, labeling, and distribution of medical devices. It includes quality control, record keeping, complaint handling, and corrective and preventive actions. Compliance with QSR is crucial to ensure consistent device quality and safety.

4. **Pre-market Approval (PMA):** Class III devices that are high-risk and novel require pre-market approval by the FDA before they can be marketed. PMA involves a comprehensive review of scientific evidence to demonstrate safety and effectiveness.

5. **Post-Market Surveillance:** Manufacturers are required to monitor and report adverse events associated with their medical devices. Post-market surveillance programs collect and analyze data on device performance, safety, and effectiveness to ensure ongoing compliance with regulations.

6. **Unique Device Identification (UDI):** UDI is a system that assigns unique identifiers to medical devices to enhance device traceability and facilitate post-market surveillance. UDI regulations require manufacturers to label devices with unique identifiers and maintain a UDI database for tracking and reporting purposes.

It's important for pharmaceutical and medical device manufacturers, healthcare professionals, and regulatory authorities to adhere to these regulations to ensure patient safety, product quality, and regulatory compliance. These regulations evolve to keep pace with advancements in technology, scientific knowledge, and changing healthcare needs.

Regulatory requirements for pharmaceuticals and medical devices (FDA regulations)

Regulatory requirements for pharmaceuticals and medical devices in the United States are primarily governed by the Food and Drug Administration (FDA). The FDA establishes and enforces regulations to ensure the safety, efficacy, and quality of these products. Here's an overview of the regulatory requirements set forth by the FDA:

Pharmaceutical Regulatory Requirements:

1. **New Drug Approval Process:** Pharmaceutical manufacturers must follow the FDA's new drug approval process to bring a new drug to market. This process involves pre-clinical studies, clinical trials, and the submission of a New Drug Application (NDA) containing data on safety, efficacy, and manufacturing.

2. **Current Good Manufacturing Practices (cGMP):** Pharmaceutical manufacturers must comply with cGMP regulations, which set the standards for the design, monitoring, and control of pharmaceutical manufacturing processes. These regulations cover areas such as facilities, equipment, personnel, quality control, documentation, and product labeling.

3. **Labeling and Drug Safety:** The FDA regulates pharmaceutical labeling to ensure accurate and comprehensive information is provided to healthcare professionals and patients. Labeling requirements include drug name, active ingredients, dosage forms, indications, contraindications, warnings, precautions, and instructions for use.

4. **Post-Marketing Surveillance:** Pharmaceutical companies are required to conduct post-marketing surveillance to monitor the safety and efficacy of drugs once they are on the market. Adverse events reporting, post-marketing studies, and label updates based on new safety information are essential components of post-marketing surveillance.

Medical Device Regulatory Requirements:

1. **Device Classification:** The FDA classifies medical devices into different categories based on risk. Class I devices are low-risk, while Class II and Class III devices have higher risk levels. Each classification is subject to specific regulatory requirements, with Class III devices being subject to the most stringent controls.

2. **Quality System Regulation (QSR):** The FDA's QSR sets the requirements for the design, manufacturing, packaging, labeling, and distribution of medical devices. QSR covers areas such as design controls, process controls, purchasing controls, complaint handling, corrective and preventive actions, and record-keeping.

3. **Pre-market Notification (510(k)):** Most Class II medical devices require a 510(k) submission to the FDA. This process demonstrates that the device is substantially equivalent to a legally marketed device and is safe and effective for its intended use.

4. **Pre-market Approval (PMA):** Class III devices, which are high-risk or novel, require a PMA submission to the FDA. This comprehensive review process assesses scientific evidence to determine the safety and effectiveness of the device.

5. **Unique Device Identification (UDI):** The FDA mandates the use of Unique Device Identification (UDI) system to identify and track medical devices throughout their lifecycle. Manufacturers must assign unique identifiers to their devices and provide UDI-related information on device labels and in a UDI database.

It's important for pharmaceutical and medical device manufacturers to comply with these regulatory requirements to ensure patient safety, product quality, and regulatory compliance. The FDA provides guidance documents, regulations, and inspections to enforce compliance with these requirements and protect public health.

Drug Approval Processes and Post-marketing Surveillance

Drug Approval Processes:

1. **Investigational New Drug (IND) Application:** Before conducting clinical trials, pharmaceutical companies must submit an IND application to the FDA. This application includes pre-clinical data and plans for clinical trials, demonstrating the drug's safety and potential efficacy. The FDA reviews the IND to ensure the proposed clinical trials meet ethical and safety standards.

2. **Clinical Trials:** Pharmaceutical companies conduct three phases of clinical trials to gather data on a drug's safety, efficacy, dosage, and potential side effects. Phase I involves a small group of healthy volunteers, Phase II expands to a larger group of patients, and Phase III involves a larger patient population to confirm effectiveness and monitor adverse reactions.

3. **New Drug Application (NDA):** After successful completion of clinical trials, pharmaceutical companies submit an NDA to the FDA. The NDA includes comprehensive data on the drug's efficacy and safety, manufacturing processes, labeling, and proposed use. The FDA reviews the NDA to evaluate the drug's benefits and risks.

4. **FDA Review and Approval:** The FDA reviews the NDA submission, assessing the drug's safety, effectiveness, and quality. This review process involves evaluating clinical trial data, manufacturing processes, labeling, and proposed use. If the FDA approves the NDA, the drug can be marketed and distributed for its approved indications.

Post-Marketing Surveillance:

1. **Adverse Event Reporting:** Pharmaceutical companies are required to monitor and report adverse events associated with their drugs to the FDA. This includes any unexpected side effects, medication errors, or quality issues. Healthcare professionals and patients can also report adverse events directly to the FDA through the MedWatch program.

2. **Post-Marketing Studies:** The FDA may require pharmaceutical companies to conduct post-marketing studies to gather additional data on the drug's safety and effectiveness. These studies may focus on specific patient populations, long-term effects, or rare adverse events not captured during clinical trials.

3. **Risk Evaluation and Mitigation Strategies (REMS):** In certain cases, the FDA may require REMS for drugs with known risks or safety concerns. REMS programs ensure safe and appropriate use of the drug by implementing specific actions, such as additional training for healthcare professionals or patient monitoring.

4. **Labeling Updates:** As new safety information becomes available, pharmaceutical companies must update their drug labeling to reflect any necessary changes. This includes adding new warnings, precautions, dosage

adjustments, or contraindications based on post-marketing surveillance and new clinical data.

5. **Ongoing Safety Monitoring:** The FDA continues to monitor drug safety even after approval. This includes analyzing adverse event reports, conducting safety reviews, and collaborating with healthcare professionals, patients, and manufacturers to ensure the ongoing safety of marketed drugs.

The drug approval process and post-marketing surveillance are designed to assess the safety and effectiveness of drugs before and after they enter the market. These processes aim to protect public health by ensuring that drugs are thoroughly evaluated, monitored for adverse events, and labeled appropriately to guide safe and effective use.

Medical Device Classification and Pre-market Clearance

Medical devices are classified into different categories based on their risk and intended use. The classification of medical devices determines the regulatory pathway and requirements for pre-market clearance. In the United States, the classification system and pre-market clearance processes are overseen by the Food and Drug Administration (FDA). Here's an overview of medical device classification and pre-market clearance:

Medical Device Classification:

1. **Class I Devices:** Class I devices are considered low-risk and are subject to the least regulatory control. Examples include tongue depressors, bandages, and elastic bandages. Most Class I devices are exempt from pre-market submission requirements, but they still need to comply with General Controls, including labeling, good manufacturing practices, and adverse event reporting.

2. **Class II Devices:** Class II devices pose moderate risk to patients and require more stringent regulatory controls. Examples include powered wheelchairs, infusion pumps, and certain diagnostic tests. Most Class II devices require a pre-market notification, known as a 510(k) submission, to demonstrate substantial equivalence to a legally marketed device.

3. **Class III Devices:** Class III devices are considered high-risk and are subject to the most rigorous regulatory controls. Examples include implantable

pacemakers, certain life-supporting devices, and novel technologies. Class III devices require a pre-market approval (PMA) application, which includes extensive scientific evidence demonstrating safety and effectiveness.

Pre-Market Clearance:

1. **510(k) Pre-Market Notification:** For Class II devices, manufacturers must submit a 510(k) pre-market notification to the FDA. The purpose of the 510(k) submission is to demonstrate that the new device is substantially equivalent to a predicate device that is already legally marketed in the United States. The FDA reviews the submission and determines whether the device can be cleared for commercial distribution.

2. **Pre-market Approval (PMA):** Class III devices, which are high-risk or novel technologies, require a PMA application. The PMA process involves providing scientific evidence, including clinical data, to demonstrate the device's safety and effectiveness. The FDA reviews the PMA application and determines whether the device can be approved for marketing and distribution.

3. **De Novo Classification:** For novel devices that do not have a predicate device to compare with, manufacturers can submit a de novo classification request. De novo classification is a pathway for low to moderate-risk devices that have not been previously classified. The FDA evaluates the device's safety and effectiveness and determines the appropriate regulatory controls.

4. **Humanitarian Use Device (HUD):** HUD designation is available for devices intended to treat or diagnose rare diseases or conditions affecting fewer than 8,000 individuals in the United States per year. HUDs require a humanitarian device exemption (HDE) application, which includes limited clinical data and evidence of safety and probable benefit.

The pre-market clearance processes aim to ensure the safety and effectiveness of medical devices before they are made available to patients and healthcare providers. Manufacturers must demonstrate compliance with relevant regulatory requirements, including performance testing, labeling, manufacturing controls, and clinical data, depending on the device's classification. The FDA's evaluation and clearance or approval provide assurance to patients and healthcare professionals regarding the device's quality and safety.

Ensuring Product Safety, Labeling, and Advertising Compliance

Ensuring product safety, labeling, and advertising compliance is critical for pharmaceuticals and medical devices to protect public health, provide accurate information to healthcare professionals and patients, and maintain regulatory compliance. Here are key strategies to ensure safety, labeling, and advertising compliance:

Product Safety:

1. **Adherence to Good Manufacturing Practices (GMP):** Follow GMP regulations to ensure the quality, safety, and consistency of pharmaceuticals and medical devices throughout the manufacturing process. Implement robust quality control systems, conduct regular inspections, and maintain documentation to demonstrate compliance with GMP requirements.

2. **Risk Assessment and Management:** Conduct thorough risk assessments to identify potential hazards and risks associated with pharmaceuticals and medical devices. Implement risk management strategies to mitigate and minimize identified risks, including proper design controls, testing, and monitoring throughout the product lifecycle.

3. **Post-Market Surveillance:** Establish systems to monitor product performance, adverse events, and safety concerns after the product is on the market. Promptly investigate and address any safety issues or unexpected adverse events. Maintain a comprehensive adverse event reporting system and comply with reporting obligations to regulatory authorities.

Labeling Compliance:

1. **FDA Labeling Requirements:** Familiarize yourself with the FDA regulations and guidelines for product labeling. Ensure that labeling content, including package inserts, patient information leaflets, and product labels, accurately and clearly convey the appropriate information, such as indications, contraindications, warnings, precautions, dosage instructions, and storage conditions.

2. **Product Identification and UDI:** For medical devices, comply with Unique Device Identification (UDI) requirements by assigning and labeling products

with unique identifiers. This allows for traceability, facilitates post-market surveillance, and supports accurate and efficient product identification.

3. **Labeling Reviews and Updates:** Establish processes for reviewing and updating product labeling as necessary. Regularly assess labeling content to ensure it remains up to date, accurate, and compliant with changing regulatory requirements. Monitor scientific advancements and safety information to make any necessary labeling revisions promptly.

Advertising Compliance:

1. **FDA and FTC Regulations:** Comply with FDA and Federal Trade Commission (FTC) regulations regarding advertising and promotion of pharmaceuticals and medical devices. Ensure that advertising materials, including websites, brochures, and promotional campaigns, are accurate, truthful, and not misleading. Avoid making unsupported claims, off-label promotions, or exaggerated statements.

2. **Substantiation of Claims:** Ensure that all claims made in advertising materials are supported by scientific evidence, clinical data, or appropriate regulatory approvals. Maintain documentation to substantiate the claims made and ensure they are consistent with the approved indications or uses.

3. **Promotional Review Process:** Implement a robust promotional review process to ensure all advertising and promotional materials undergo thorough internal review and approval. Involve cross-functional teams, including regulatory, legal, and marketing, to assess compliance with applicable regulations and guidelines.

4. **Adverse Event Reporting:** Implement systems to capture and report any adverse events related to product advertising. Maintain records of reported adverse events and promptly address any concerns or issues identified during the monitoring process.

Regular training and education of employees on product safety, labeling requirements, and advertising compliance are essential. Ensure that employees understand their roles and responsibilities, and provide ongoing guidance and updates regarding regulatory requirements and industry best practices. Establish a culture of compliance and implement effective quality management systems to support ongoing monitoring and improvement efforts.

Chapter 07

Compliance Challenges in Research and Clinical Trials

Compliance challenges in research and clinical trials can arise due to the complex and regulated nature of these activities. The following are some common compliance challenges faced in research and clinical trials:

1. **Ethical Considerations:** Ensuring ethical compliance is crucial in research and clinical trials. Challenges may include obtaining informed consent from participants, protecting participant rights and privacy, and maintaining confidentiality of sensitive data. Balancing the benefits and risks of the study and ensuring the well-being of participants can be challenging.

2. **Regulatory Compliance:** Clinical trials are subject to various regulations and guidelines from regulatory authorities such as the FDA or the International Council for Harmonization of Technical Requirements for Pharmaceuticals for Human Use (ICH). Compliance challenges may include obtaining necessary regulatory approvals, adhering to protocol requirements, and meeting reporting obligations.

3. **Data Integrity and Management:** Maintaining accurate and reliable data throughout the research and clinical trial process is critical. Compliance challenges include ensuring data integrity, protecting against data manipulation or falsification, and maintaining proper documentation and record-keeping practices.

4. **Institutional Review Board (IRB) Approval:** Research involving human participants requires review and approval from an IRB. Challenges can arise in obtaining timely and consistent IRB approval, addressing concerns raised by the IRB, and ensuring ongoing compliance with IRB requirements throughout the study.

5. **Safety Reporting and Adverse Event Monitoring:** Reporting and monitoring participant safety and adverse events are essential in clinical trials. Challenges may include timely identification, documentation, and reporting of adverse events, ensuring proper risk management, and implementing appropriate safety monitoring protocols.

6. **Financial Disclosure and Conflict of Interest:** Researchers and investigators may have financial interests or conflicts of interest that need to be disclosed and managed. Compliance challenges include accurately disclosing financial relationships, implementing conflict of interest policies, and ensuring transparency in reporting financial interests.

7. **Quality Assurance and Quality Control:** Maintaining high-quality research and trial processes is crucial for compliance. Challenges include implementing effective quality assurance and quality control mechanisms, conducting regular audits, and addressing any non-compliance or deviations from protocols or regulations.

8. **International Collaboration and Compliance:** Research and clinical trials often involve international collaborations, leading to additional compliance challenges. Ensuring compliance with regulations and guidelines from multiple jurisdictions, addressing cultural and ethical differences, and harmonizing processes and documentation across countries can be complex.

To address these compliance challenges, organizations involved in research and clinical trials should establish robust compliance programs, provide ongoing training to research staff, engage in proactive risk assessment and management, and foster a culture of compliance. Collaboration with regulatory authorities, ethics committees, and IRBs is essential to stay updated on regulations and guidelines and to address compliance issues effectively.

Ethical Considerations in Research and Clinical Trials

Ethical considerations in research and clinical trials are paramount to protect the rights, welfare, and well-being of participants. Adhering to ethical principles ensures that research is conducted with integrity, transparency, and respect for the dignity and autonomy of individuals. Here are key ethical considerations in research and clinical trials (Table 7.1):

▼ **Table 7.1:** Common Compliance Challenges in Research and Clinical Trials

Compliance Challenge	Description
Informed Consent Issues	Challenges related to obtaining informed consent from participants, ensuring understanding and voluntariness.
Protocol Deviations	Instances where the study protocol is not followed as intended, leading to non-compliance with study procedures.
Data Integrity and Management	Challenges in maintaining accurate and complete data, ensuring proper data collection, storage, and security.
Financial Conflicts of Interest	Issues related to financial interests that may compromise objectivity, such as sponsor or investigator conflicts.
Investigational Product Handling	Compliance challenges in the proper handling, storage, and administration of investigational products.

1. **Informed Consent:** Participants must provide voluntary and informed consent before participating in research. This includes providing clear and understandable information about the study purpose, procedures, potential risks and benefits, alternatives, and the right to withdraw at any time without repercussions. Informed consent ensures that participants make autonomous decisions based on accurate information.

2. **Beneficence and Non-maleficence:** Researchers have an ethical obligation to maximize benefits and minimize harm to participants. The potential benefits of the study should outweigh the potential risks. Safeguards should be in place to protect participants from physical, psychological, or social harm. Regular monitoring and assessment of participant well-being are essential.

3. **Privacy and Confidentiality:** Participants' privacy rights should be respected, and their personal information must be kept confidential. Researchers should implement appropriate measures to protect participant data and ensure that information is disclosed only as required by law or with explicit consent. Anonymity and confidentiality should be maintained during data collection, analysis, and dissemination.

4. **Equitable Participant Selection:** Participants should be selected in a fair and unbiased manner, without discrimination or undue influence. Recruitment

strategies should avoid targeting vulnerable populations and strive for inclusivity and diversity. The benefits and burdens of participation should be distributed fairly among different groups.

5. **Research Integrity:** Researchers must adhere to high standards of scientific integrity, ensuring accurate reporting of methods, results, and conclusions. Falsification, fabrication, or selective reporting of data should be strictly prohibited. Transparency, openness, and reproducibility of research findings are crucial for the advancement of knowledge and trust in the research community.

6. **Conflict of Interest:** Researchers should disclose and manage any potential conflicts of interest that may compromise the objectivity or integrity of the research. Financial, professional, or personal relationships that could bias the research process or outcomes should be disclosed and appropriately managed to maintain transparency and trust.

7. **Continuing Ethical Review:** Ethical oversight and review should continue throughout the research process. Institutional Review Boards (IRBs) or Ethics Committees play a critical role in evaluating research proposals, monitoring ongoing studies, and ensuring compliance with ethical guidelines. Regular ethical reviews and oversight help to identify and address emerging ethical concerns.

8. **Publication and Dissemination:** Findings from research should be disseminated in a timely and transparent manner. Researchers have an ethical responsibility to report results accurately, honestly, and without selective reporting. Sharing research findings contributes to the collective knowledge and informs future research and clinical practices.

Adhering to ethical considerations is essential to maintain the integrity and trustworthiness of research and clinical trials. Researchers and institutions must follow ethical guidelines, obtain appropriate approvals, conduct thorough informed consent processes, and prioritize participant welfare throughout the research journey.

Compliance with Human Subjects Protection Regulations (IRB, Common Rule)

Compliance with human subjects protection regulations is crucial to ensure the ethical and responsible conduct of research involving human participants (Table 7.2). Two key regulations that govern human subjects protection in the United States are the Institutional Review Board (IRB) oversight and the Common Rule. Here's an overview of compliance with these regulations:

1. **Institutional Review Board (IRB):**

   - An IRB is an independent committee responsible for reviewing, approving, and overseeing research involving human participants. IRBs ensure that research complies with ethical principles and regulatory requirements.

   - Compliance involves submitting research protocols to the IRB for review and obtaining IRB approval before initiating the study.

   - Researchers must provide comprehensive information about the study, including the purpose, procedures, potential risks and benefits, informed consent process, and participant protection measures.

   - IRBs evaluate the ethical aspects of the research, including participant selection, informed consent process, privacy and confidentiality, risks and benefits, and researcher conflicts of interest.

   - Compliance also involves ongoing reporting of study progress, any protocol modifications, and adverse events to the IRB.

   - Researchers and institutions must follow the IRB's recommendations and maintain ongoing communication and cooperation with the IRB throughout the study.

2. **Common Rule:**

   - The Common Rule is a federal policy that provides ethical standards and regulations for the protection of human subjects in research.

   - Compliance involves ensuring that research studies funded or conducted by federal departments and agencies adhere to the Common Rule requirements.

   - Key elements of compliance include informed consent, minimization of risks, selection of participants, privacy and confidentiality protection, and fair and equitable recruitment practices.

   - Compliance also requires the creation and maintenance of an assurance of compliance with the Common Rule by institutions conducting research.

   - The Common Rule emphasizes transparency, accountability, and ongoing monitoring of research activities to protect the rights and welfare of human subjects.

To ensure compliance with human subjects protection regulations:

1. **Educate and Train:** Researchers, study coordinators, and other relevant personnel should receive training on human subjects protection,

ethical principles, and regulatory requirements. This ensures a clear understanding of the responsibilities and obligations associated with research involving human participants.

2. **Develop Comprehensive Protocols:** Researchers should develop well-designed research protocols that address ethical considerations, informed consent procedures, participant selection criteria, privacy and confidentiality protection, and risk mitigation strategies. Protocols should align with IRB and Common Rule requirements.

3. **Engage with the IRB:** Establish open lines of communication with the IRB, seek their guidance during protocol development, and promptly address any concerns or feedback. Provide timely updates on study progress, modifications, and adverse events as required by the IRB.

4. **Maintain Accurate Documentation:** Keep thorough and accurate records of the research study, including protocol versions, informed consent documents, IRB correspondence, adverse event reports, and any other relevant documentation. Documentation should be easily accessible and organized to demonstrate compliance with human subjects protection regulations.

5. **Regular Monitoring and Auditing:** Conduct regular internal monitoring and auditing of research activities to ensure compliance with IRB and Common Rule requirements. Identify any potential deviations, non-compliance, or areas for improvement and implement corrective actions promptly.

6. **Stay Updated:** Stay informed about changes in IRB policies, guidelines, and regulatory requirements. Monitor updates to the Common Rule and other relevant regulations to ensure ongoing compliance with evolving standards.

▼ **Table 7.2:** Strategies for Addressing Compliance Challenges

Compliance Challenge	Strategies
Informed Consent Issues	Provide comprehensive participant education, use plain language, ensure adequate time for decision-making.
Protocol Deviations	Implement robust monitoring and oversight mechanisms, conduct regular site visits and audits.
Data Integrity and Management	Implement data management plans, ensure proper training and documentation of data handling procedures.

Compliance Challenge	Strategies
Financial Conflicts of Interest	Implement disclosure policies, establish independent review committees, and monitor financial relationships.
Investigational Product Handling	Develop and implement standard operating procedures (SOPs) for product storage, handling, and administration.

Compliance with human subjects protection regulations demonstrates a commitment to participant welfare, ethical conduct, and responsible research practices. Collaboration with IRBs and adherence to the Common Rule fosters trust, ensures participant rights are respected, and advances the integrity of research involving human subjects.

Informed Consent and Privacy Concerns in Research

Informed consent and privacy concerns are significant considerations in research involving human participants. Respecting participant autonomy, safeguarding their privacy, and ensuring the confidentiality of their personal information are crucial ethical and legal obligations. Here's an overview of these concerns in research:

1. **Informed Consent:**

   - Informed consent is the process by which participants voluntarily and comprehensively provide their consent to participate in research.

   - Researchers must provide clear and understandable information about the study purpose, procedures, potential risks and benefits, alternative options, and the right to withdraw at any time without consequences.

   - Participants should have the opportunity to ask questions, receive clarifications, and make an informed decision about their participation.

   - Informed consent should be obtained in a culturally sensitive manner and tailored to the participant's level of understanding.

   - Compliance involves documenting the informed consent process, ensuring participant comprehension, and obtaining signed consent forms.

- Ongoing communication and the ability to re-consent are important if any changes to the research occur that might affect participant rights or risks.

2. **Privacy Concerns:**

- Privacy concerns focus on protecting participants' personal information and preventing unauthorized access or disclosure.

- Researchers should implement measures to ensure participant privacy, such as collecting and storing data securely, using de-identification techniques when possible, and limiting access to personal information.

- Compliance with privacy regulations, such as the Health Insurance Portability and Accountability Act (HIPAA) in the United States, is essential in research involving protected health information.

- Researchers should communicate privacy policies and inform participants about how their data will be collected, used, stored, and shared.

- Data sharing practices should adhere to applicable regulations and guidelines, and participants' identities should be anonymized or pseudonymized whenever possible.

3. **Confidentiality:**

- Confidentiality ensures that participants' information remains private and is not disclosed to unauthorized individuals or entities.

- Researchers should establish protocols to maintain confidentiality, including secure data storage, limited access to personal information, and encryption or password protection of digital data.

- Compliance requires obtaining participants' consent for the collection, use, and storage of their personal information and implementing necessary safeguards to prevent unauthorized access or disclosure.

- Researchers should clearly communicate confidentiality measures to participants and provide assurances that their information will be protected.

4. **Data Sharing and Research Transparency:**

- Data sharing practices should balance participant privacy with the benefits of sharing research data for scientific advancement.

- Compliance involves ensuring that data sharing policies are clearly communicated to participants during the informed consent process.

- Researchers should consider obtaining separate consent for data sharing, specify the types of data to be shared, describe any data sharing agreements, and provide options for participants to restrict or revoke consent for data sharing.

Addressing informed consent and privacy concerns requires adherence to ethical guidelines, regulations, and best practices, as well as ongoing communication and transparency with participants. Researchers should prioritize participant autonomy, privacy, and confidentiality throughout the research process and take proactive measures to protect personal information. Collaboration with institutional review boards (IRBs) and compliance with applicable privacy regulations are vital to ensure ethical and legal compliance in research.

Monitoring and Auditing Clinical Trials for Compliance

Monitoring and auditing clinical trials for compliance is essential to ensure that research is conducted in accordance with ethical principles, regulatory requirements, and protocol specifications. These processes help identify deviations, errors, or non-compliance issues, allowing for corrective actions to be implemented promptly. Here's an overview of monitoring and auditing in clinical trials:

1. **Monitoring:**

   - Monitoring involves the ongoing assessment and oversight of a clinical trial to ensure compliance with ethical, regulatory, and protocol requirements.

   - Monitoring can be conducted by the sponsor, contract research organizations (CROs), or independent monitors.

   - Key aspects of monitoring include verifying participant eligibility, informed consent process, adherence to the study protocol, accurate and timely data collection, and adverse event reporting.

   - Monitoring visits can be conducted on-site at the study site (on-site monitoring) or remotely through centralized data monitoring and source data verification (remote monitoring).

- Monitoring activities may include reviewing study documents, source data, participant records, regulatory compliance, investigator site file (ISF), and ensuring adherence to Good Clinical Practice (GCP) guidelines.

- Monitoring findings and observations should be documented, and any identified issues or non-compliance should be addressed through corrective and preventive actions.

2. **Auditing:**

- Auditing involves independent and systematic examinations of clinical trial processes, procedures, and data to ensure compliance, accuracy, and reliability.

- Audits can be conducted by internal audit teams within the sponsor or independent external auditors.

- Audits may encompass various aspects of the clinical trial, including investigator sites, CROs, data management, pharmacovigilance, quality systems, and compliance with regulatory requirements.

- Auditing can be conducted during the trial (ongoing audits) or after the trial's completion (post-trial audits).

- Audits may involve document reviews, site visits, interviews with investigators and study staff, data verification, and assessment of compliance with GCP and applicable regulations.

- Audit findings and recommendations should be documented, and appropriate actions should be taken to address any identified issues or non-compliance.

3. **Risk-Based Monitoring:**

- Risk-based monitoring (RBM) is an approach that focuses monitoring efforts on areas with the highest risk to participant safety, data integrity, and study quality.

- RBM utilizes a combination of centralized data monitoring, targeted on-site monitoring, and remote monitoring techniques.

- RBM involves assessing risks, developing a monitoring plan, and adapting monitoring activities based on ongoing risk assessment throughout the trial.

- The use of RBM allows for more efficient and effective allocation of monitoring resources, targeting critical areas that require closer scrutiny.

4. **Quality Assurance (QA):**

- Quality assurance involves implementing processes and systems to ensure that clinical trials are conducted in compliance with applicable regulations, guidelines, and quality standards.

- QA activities include establishing quality management systems, standard operating procedures (SOPs), and document control.

- QA ensures that appropriate training is provided to investigators and study staff, and that processes are in place for data management, adverse event reporting, and protocol compliance.

- QA functions may include conducting internal audits, assessing compliance with SOPs, overseeing corrective and preventive actions, and maintaining compliance with GCP and regulatory requirements.

Monitoring and auditing are integral parts of ensuring compliance and the integrity of clinical trials. These processes help identify and address issues early, promote data accuracy and participant safety, and contribute to the overall quality of clinical research. Collaboration among sponsors, investigators, study staff, and regulatory authorities is essential to establish effective monitoring and auditing practices in clinical trials.

Compliance in a Changing Healthcare Landscape

Compliance in a changing healthcare landscape is a critical aspect for healthcare organizations to ensure adherence to evolving regulations, address emerging risks, and adapt to new models of care delivery. This involves proactively managing compliance programs, staying updated with regulatory changes, and fostering a culture of compliance throughout the organization. Here are some key considerations for compliance in a changing healthcare landscape:

1. **Regulatory Awareness:** Healthcare organizations must stay vigilant about regulatory changes and updates. This includes monitoring updates from regulatory bodies such as the Centers for Medicare and Medicaid Services (CMS), the Office of Inspector General (OIG), and other relevant authorities. Regularly reviewing and interpreting new regulations helps compliance professionals understand the implications for their organization and take necessary steps to ensure compliance.

2. **Compliance Program Evaluation:** Compliance programs should be periodically evaluated to assess their effectiveness in the changing healthcare landscape. This involves reviewing policies, procedures, and protocols to align them with current regulations and industry best practices. Compliance risk assessments can identify emerging risks and guide the development of mitigation strategies.

3. **Educating and Training:** Compliance education and training should be ongoing to keep employees informed about changes in regulations, industry standards, and emerging compliance risks. Training programs should address specific compliance areas relevant to the changing healthcare landscape, such as telemedicine, data privacy, and value-based care. Ensuring that employees have the knowledge and skills to navigate these changes promotes a culture of compliance.

4. **Technology and Data Security:** Healthcare organizations are increasingly relying on technology for data management, communication, and care delivery. Compliance efforts should encompass data security and privacy considerations. Implementing robust cybersecurity measures, conducting regular risk assessments, and ensuring compliance with data protection regulations (such as HIPAA) are essential to protect patient information and maintain regulatory compliance.

5. **Collaboration with Stakeholders:** Collaboration among compliance professionals, healthcare providers, legal teams, and other stakeholders is crucial in addressing compliance challenges in a changing landscape. Engaging with these stakeholders allows for a better understanding of evolving risks and helps develop effective compliance strategies. Sharing information, best practices, and lessons learned can enhance compliance efforts collectively.

6. **Ethical Decision-Making:** As the healthcare landscape evolves, ethical considerations become increasingly important. Compliance professionals should foster an ethical culture within the organization, promoting ethical decision-making at all levels. This includes addressing conflicts of interest, promoting transparency, and ensuring patient-centered care.

7. **Auditing and Monitoring:** Regular auditing and monitoring activities are essential in the changing healthcare landscape to identify compliance gaps, assess the effectiveness of controls, and detect and address non-compliance. Leveraging data analytics and technology can enhance auditing capabilities and facilitate proactive monitoring of compliance risks.

8. **Continuous Improvement:** Compliance programs should be subject to continuous improvement efforts. This involves learning from past experiences, conducting root cause analyses of compliance incidents, and implementing corrective actions to prevent recurrence. Ongoing evaluation and adjustment of compliance processes help organizations adapt to changes and ensure long-term compliance success.

Compliance in a changing healthcare landscape requires adaptability, agility, and a proactive approach. By actively monitoring regulatory changes, updating compliance programs, promoting ethical behavior, and collaborating with stakeholders, healthcare organizations can effectively navigate the challenges and maintain compliance in an ever-evolving industry.

Impact of Healthcare Reforms and Policy Changes on Regulatory Compliance

Healthcare reforms and policy changes can have a significant impact on regulatory compliance for healthcare organizations. These reforms aim to improve access to care, enhance patient outcomes, control costs, and address gaps in the healthcare system. Compliance professionals must navigate the evolving regulatory landscape and ensure their organizations remain compliant. Here are some key impacts of healthcare reforms and policy changes on regulatory compliance:

1. **Changes in Payment Models:** Reforms often introduce new payment models, such as value-based care and alternative payment models (APMs). These models shift the focus from fee-for-service to quality and value. Compliance professionals must understand the new payment methodologies, reporting requirements, and compliance obligations associated with these models. This may involve implementing new systems to track and report quality measures, ensuring accurate billing and coding practices, and monitoring compliance with specific program requirements.

2. **Increased Emphasis on Quality and Patient Outcomes:** Healthcare reforms often prioritize quality improvement and patient outcomes. Compliance professionals need to align their compliance programs with these objectives. This may involve implementing quality reporting systems, ensuring accurate documentation and reporting of clinical outcomes, and monitoring compliance with quality improvement initiatives. Compliance professionals may also be involved in activities such as conducting internal audits and risk assessments to identify areas for improvement and address gaps in quality and patient safety.

3. **Enhanced Privacy and Security Protections:** Healthcare reforms may introduce or strengthen privacy and security regulations to protect patient health information. Compliance professionals must stay updated with changes to privacy laws, such as the Health Insurance Portability and Accountability Act (HIPAA) and the General Data Protection Regulation (GDPR), and ensure their organizations' policies and practices align with these requirements. This includes implementing appropriate safeguards for data protection, conducting regular risk assessments, and addressing breaches or incidents involving patient information.

4. **Increased Focus on Fraud and Abuse Prevention:** Healthcare reforms often include provisions to combat fraud, waste, and abuse in the healthcare system. Compliance professionals must monitor changes in anti-fraud regulations, such as the False Claims Act, Anti-Kickback Statute, and Stark Law, and ensure their organizations have robust compliance programs to prevent, detect, and respond to potential violations. This may involve implementing effective internal controls, conducting regular audits, providing compliance training, and establishing mechanisms for reporting and investigating potential violations.

5. **Regulatory Reporting and Transparency:** Healthcare reforms may introduce new reporting requirements and increased transparency in healthcare. Compliance professionals must understand and comply with these reporting obligations. This may include reporting on quality measures, financial transactions, conflicts of interest, or other relevant data to regulatory authorities or public entities. Compliance professionals may need to develop or enhance systems to collect, analyze, and report the required data accurately and promptly.

6. **Changes in Reimbursement and Billing Rules:** Healthcare reforms may lead to changes in reimbursement rates, billing rules, and documentation requirements. Compliance professionals must stay updated with these changes and ensure their organizations' billing and coding practices are compliant. This may involve implementing appropriate controls to prevent billing errors, conducting regular audits of billing processes, and providing training to billing and coding staff to ensure accurate and compliant practices.

7. **Expanded Regulatory Oversight and Enforcement:** Healthcare reforms often lead to increased regulatory oversight and enforcement efforts. Compliance professionals must be aware of heightened scrutiny and ensure their organizations have robust compliance programs in place. This includes conducting internal audits, implementing effective monitoring and reporting mechanisms, and promptly addressing any identified compliance issues.

Navigating the impact of healthcare reforms and policy changes on regulatory compliance requires a proactive and adaptable approach. Compliance professionals must stay updated with regulatory updates, collaborate with stakeholders, assess and mitigate compliance risks, and continuously improve their compliance programs to align with the evolving healthcare landscape.

Evolving Technologies and their Implications for Compliance (Telemedicine, AI, Wearables)

Evolving technologies, such as telemedicine, artificial intelligence (AI), and wearables, have transformative potential in healthcare. However, these technologies also introduce new compliance considerations that must be addressed by healthcare organizations. Here are some key implications of evolving technologies for compliance:

1. **Telemedicine:**

    - Telemedicine enables remote patient consultations and care delivery through telecommunications technology.

    - Compliance considerations include adhering to licensing and credentialing requirements for healthcare providers practicing across state or international borders.

    - Ensuring privacy and security of patient information during telehealth encounters is critical, requiring compliance with data protection regulations (e.g., HIPAA).

    - Compliance professionals must address reimbursement and billing requirements specific to telemedicine services, including documenting and coding telehealth encounters accurately.

2. **Artificial Intelligence (AI):**

    - AI technologies, such as machine learning and natural language processing, are increasingly used in healthcare for diagnostics, treatment planning, and decision support.

    - Compliance considerations involve ensuring the transparency, explainability, and fairness of AI algorithms to avoid bias and discrimination in patient care.

    - Compliance professionals must address data privacy and security concerns associated with AI applications, especially when handling sensitive patient information.

    - Compliance with regulatory requirements, such as FDA regulations for AI-based medical devices, is crucial for AI technology used in clinical decision-making.

3. **Wearables and Remote Monitoring:**

- Wearable devices and remote monitoring technologies enable continuous monitoring of patient health parameters outside traditional healthcare settings.

- Compliance professionals need to address data privacy and security concerns associated with collecting, transmitting, and storing patient data from wearables and remote monitoring devices.

- Compliance with data protection regulations, such as HIPAA, is crucial when wearable devices collect and transmit patient health information.

- Compliance considerations may include ensuring accuracy and reliability of wearable device data, validating the use of wearables in clinical decision-making, and addressing patient consent and data sharing practices.

4. **Data Governance and Analytics:**

- Evolving technologies generate vast amounts of healthcare data that can be utilized for analytics and insights.

- Compliance professionals must address data governance and management practices to ensure the privacy, security, and ethical use of healthcare data.

- Compliance with data protection regulations, such as HIPAA and GDPR, is crucial when using healthcare data for research, analytics, or AI model training.

- Compliance considerations include anonymization or de-identification of patient data, securing data access and sharing, and implementing controls to prevent data breaches or unauthorized access.

5. **Interoperability and Data Exchange:**

- Evolving technologies require seamless interoperability and data exchange between different healthcare systems and devices.

- Compliance professionals must address interoperability standards and regulations to ensure the secure and standardized exchange of patient information.

- Compliance considerations include adhering to regulatory requirements, such as the CMS Interoperability and Patient Access Final Rule, which mandates the sharing of patient health information between healthcare organizations.

- Ensuring patient consent and control over the sharing of their health data is critical in the context of evolving technologies and data exchange.

Compliance professionals must proactively assess the compliance implications of evolving technologies, develop policies and procedures to address associated risks, and collaborate with stakeholders to ensure regulatory compliance. Staying updated with evolving regulations and guidelines specific to these technologies is crucial to navigate the compliance challenges presented by telemedicine, AI, wearables, and other transformative technologies in healthcare.

International Regulations and Global Compliance Challenges

International regulations and global compliance challenges are crucial considerations for healthcare organizations operating across borders or engaging in international collaborations. Compliance professionals must navigate diverse regulatory frameworks, cultural differences, and varying enforcement practices. Here are key aspects of international regulations and global compliance challenges (Table 8.1):

1. **Data Privacy and Security:** Data protection regulations vary across countries, such as the General Data Protection Regulation (GDPR) in the European Union, the Health Information Portability and Accountability Act (HIPAA) in the United States, and other country-specific data privacy laws. Compliance professionals must ensure that international data transfers comply with relevant regulations, establish data protection measures, and address cross-border data flow challenges.

2. **Anti-Corruption and Bribery Laws:** Compliance with anti-corruption laws, such as the U.S. Foreign Corrupt Practices Act (FCPA) and the UK Bribery Act, is essential for global operations. Compliance professionals should implement anti-corruption policies and procedures, conduct due diligence on business partners and third-party vendors, and provide training to employees on anti-corruption practices.

3. **Trade Compliance and Export Controls:** Healthcare organizations involved in the international distribution of medical products or technologies must comply with trade compliance regulations, export controls, and sanctions. Compliance professionals should understand the export control laws of different countries, screen transactions against restricted party lists, and implement appropriate controls to prevent illegal exports.

4. **Cross-Cultural Compliance:** Cultural differences and varying ethical standards across countries present compliance challenges. Compliance professionals must adapt compliance programs to local cultural norms, language, and business practices. This includes tailoring training and communication materials, understanding local regulatory requirements, and promoting ethical behavior and integrity in international operations.

5. **Transparency and Reporting:** Transparency and reporting requirements differ globally, such as the Sunshine Act in the United States, which mandates the disclosure of financial relationships with healthcare professionals. Compliance professionals should stay informed about local transparency regulations, track reporting obligations, and ensure accurate and timely reporting of relevant data.

6. **Global Supply Chain Compliance:** Healthcare organizations with global supply chains face compliance challenges related to supplier due diligence, product quality, counterfeit products, and ethical sourcing practices. Compliance professionals should implement supplier compliance programs, conduct audits of suppliers, and ensure adherence to quality standards and ethical guidelines throughout the supply chain.

7. **Local Licensing and Regulatory Requirements:** Healthcare organizations expanding globally must navigate diverse licensing and regulatory requirements across jurisdictions. Compliance professionals should ensure compliance with local regulations, obtain necessary licenses and permits, and establish processes to monitor changes in regulatory environments.

8. **Enforcement and Legal Jurisdiction:** Legal enforcement practices and the availability of remedies for non-compliance vary across countries. Compliance professionals should understand the legal frameworks and jurisdictional issues relevant to their global operations. Collaboration with legal counsel, local experts, and engaging in dialogs with regulatory authorities is important to navigate enforcement challenges.

▼ **Table 8.1:** Compliance Challenges in a Changing Landscape

Compliance Challenge	Description
Evolving Regulatory Environment	Challenges in keeping up with changing regulations and ensuring compliance with new requirements.
Technology Adoption and Security	Addressing the compliance implications of adopting new technologies while ensuring data security.
Transitioning Payment Models	Navigating the transition from traditional fee-for-service to value-based payment models.
Data Privacy and Cybersecurity	Protecting patient data and ensuring compliance with privacy regulations in an increasingly digital healthcare environment.

Addressing international regulations and global compliance challenges requires a proactive and adaptive approach. Compliance professionals should engage in continuous learning, stay updated with international laws and regulations, foster cross-functional collaborations, and establish effective compliance programs tailored to local requirements. Collaboration with local partners and leveraging external expertise can help navigate the complexities of global compliance.

Strategies for Staying Updated with Regulatory Changes

Staying updated with regulatory changes is crucial for compliance professionals to effectively navigate the evolving regulatory landscape. Here are some strategies to help stay abreast of regulatory changes:

1. **Regulatory Monitoring Services:** Subscribe to regulatory monitoring services, which provide updates on relevant regulations and changes in the legal landscape. These services can deliver regular email alerts or newsletters that highlight key regulatory developments in your industry or region.

2. **Government Websites and Regulatory Agencies:** Regularly visit government websites and regulatory agency portals that oversee the industry or sector you operate in. These websites often provide updated information on regulations, guidance documents, and announcements of regulatory changes. Subscribe to mailing lists or RSS feeds offered by these agencies to receive notifications directly.

3. **Industry Associations and Trade Organizations:** Join industry associations and trade organizations that focus on compliance and regulatory matters in your sector. These organizations often provide valuable resources, newsletters, webinars, and events that address regulatory changes. They may also offer networking opportunities with peers and experts in the field.

4. **Networking and Professional Communities:** Engage in networking activities and participate in professional communities related to compliance and regulatory affairs. Attending industry conferences, seminars, and workshops can provide valuable insights into regulatory changes and compliance best practices. Engaging with peers through online forums, discussion groups, and social media platforms can also facilitate the exchange of knowledge and information.

5. **Regulatory Impact Assessments:** Conduct regular regulatory impact assessments to evaluate the potential impact of regulatory changes on your organization. This involves reviewing proposed regulations, guidance documents, and policy statements to understand how they may affect your compliance program and operations. Engage relevant stakeholders within your organization to gather insights and perspectives on the potential impact.

6. **Collaboration with Legal Counsel:** Work closely with your organization's legal counsel to understand the implications of regulatory changes. Regularly communicate with them to receive updates on legal developments and seek their guidance on compliance matters. Legal counsel can help interpret complex regulatory requirements and provide advice on compliance strategies.

7. **Engagement with Regulatory Authorities:** Foster relationships and engage in dialogue with regulatory authorities relevant to your industry. Attend public meetings, comment on proposed regulations, and participate in industry working groups or advisory committees. Building a rapport with regulators can provide valuable insights into upcoming regulatory changes and help shape policy discussions.

8. **Continuing Education and Training:** Invest in continuous education and professional development programs for yourself and your compliance team. Attend webinars, seminars, and training sessions offered by reputable organizations specializing in regulatory compliance. Certifications and professional courses in compliance can enhance your knowledge and skills in navigating regulatory changes.

9. **Internal Communication and Collaboration:** Establish effective communication channels within your organization to share regulatory updates. Collaborate with relevant departments, such as legal, risk management, and operations, to gather insights and ensure a coordinated approach to compliance. Regularly communicate regulatory changes to key stakeholders and conduct training sessions to raise awareness within the organization.

By employing these strategies, compliance professionals can stay updated with regulatory changes, anticipate potential compliance challenges, and proactively adapt their compliance programs to ensure ongoing regulatory compliance.

Chapter 09

Training and Education for Compliance

Training and education are vital components of a successful compliance program, helping to ensure that employees and stakeholders understand their compliance obligations and can effectively navigate regulatory requirements. Here are some key aspects to consider regarding training and education for compliance:

1. **Training Needs Assessment:** Conduct a thorough assessment to identify the specific compliance training needs within your organization. Assess the roles and responsibilities of employees, the regulatory landscape, and any areas of potential compliance risk. This assessment will help tailor training programs to address the specific needs of different departments and individuals.

2. **Compliance Training Program Design:** Develop a comprehensive compliance training program that aligns with the organization's compliance objectives and regulatory requirements. Consider utilizing a variety of training methods such as in-person workshops, online modules, webinars, or a combination of these approaches. The program should be engaging, interactive, and regularly updated to reflect changes in regulations and compliance best practices.

3. **Employee Training:** Provide training to all employees, irrespective of their roles, to ensure a baseline understanding of compliance expectations. Cover topics such as regulatory requirements, code of conduct, reporting mechanisms, and consequences of non-compliance. Use real-life scenarios and case studies to illustrate compliance principles and encourage active participation.

4. **Role-Specific Training:** Tailor training programs to the specific roles and responsibilities of employees. Different departments and positions may have

unique compliance considerations. Provide targeted training that addresses the compliance challenges faced by healthcare providers, billing and coding staff, researchers, administrators, and other relevant roles. This ensures that employees understand how compliance principles apply to their specific functions.

5. **Leadership Training:** Offer specialized compliance training for executives, managers, and supervisors to emphasize their role in promoting a culture of compliance. Focus on ethical decision-making, setting the right tone from the top, and creating an environment where compliance is prioritized. Leadership training should provide practical guidance on handling compliance issues, reporting obligations, and supporting employees in their compliance efforts.

6. **Vendor and Third-Party Training:** Extend compliance training to vendors, contractors, and other external stakeholders who have access to sensitive data or are involved in critical compliance processes. Ensure that contracts and agreements include provisions for compliance training, monitoring, and auditing. Offer training programs tailored to the specific needs of these external parties to ensure alignment with your organization's compliance standards.

7. **Ongoing Training and Education:** Compliance training should not be a one-time event but an ongoing process. Stay updated with regulatory changes, emerging risks, and industry best practices. Provide regular updates and refresher training to employees to reinforce compliance principles and address any new developments. Encourage continuous learning through webinars, newsletters, and access to relevant compliance resources.

8. **Evaluation and Measurement:** Regularly assess the effectiveness of your compliance training and education programs. Use assessments, quizzes, or simulations to evaluate knowledge retention and application of compliance principles. Collect feedback from trainees to identify areas for improvement and ensure that training programs are meeting their objectives. Use data and metrics to measure the impact of training efforts on compliance outcomes.

By implementing a comprehensive and well-designed training and education program, healthcare organizations can promote a culture of compliance, enhance employee understanding of regulatory requirements, and mitigate compliance risks effectively. Continuous evaluation and improvement of training initiatives will ensure that compliance remains a priority within the organization.

Importance of Training and Education in Promoting Compliance

Training and education play a crucial role in promoting compliance within healthcare organizations. Here are some key reasons why training and education are important in promoting compliance (Figure 9.1):

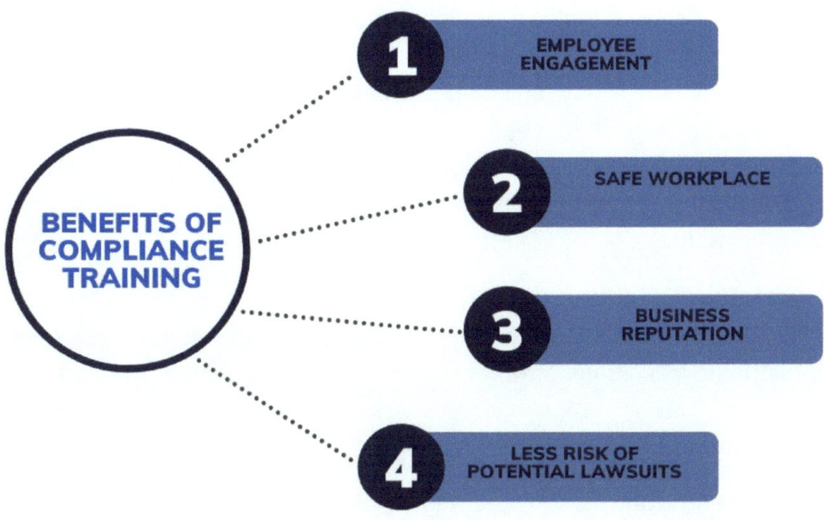

▼ **Figure 9.1:** Benefits of Compliance Training and Education

1. **Awareness and Understanding:** Training and education programs create awareness among employees about the importance of compliance, the regulatory requirements that apply to their roles, and the potential consequences of non-compliance. By increasing awareness and understanding, employees are more likely to recognize compliance risks and make informed decisions that align with regulatory expectations.

2. **Knowledge of Regulatory Requirements:** Compliance training ensures that employees have a clear understanding of the specific regulatory requirements that apply to their work. This includes laws, regulations, industry standards, and internal policies. When employees are knowledgeable about these requirements, they can apply them

appropriately in their day-to-day activities, reducing the risk of non-compliance.

3. **Risk Identification and Mitigation:** Training programs equip employees with the skills to identify and assess compliance risks within their areas of responsibility. By understanding the potential risks, employees can take proactive measures to mitigate them and prevent compliance violations. This includes recognizing red flags, reporting concerns, and seeking guidance when faced with uncertain situations.

4. **Ethical Decision-Making:** Training and education foster ethical decision-making by providing employees with guidance on ethical principles and dilemmas they may encounter. Through case studies, discussions, and interactive exercises, employees can develop their ethical reasoning skills, enabling them to make decisions that prioritize compliance and ethical behavior.

5. **Behavioral Change and Cultural Transformation:** Effective training programs can contribute to a cultural transformation within an organization. By emphasizing the importance of compliance, promoting ethical behavior, and setting expectations for compliance, training can shape the organization's culture. This, in turn, encourages a shared commitment to compliance and establishes a foundation for a strong compliance culture.

6. **Risk Reduction and Legal Protection:** Comprehensive training and education programs reduce the likelihood of compliance violations and associated legal issues. When employees are well-trained, they are more likely to adhere to regulatory requirements, follow internal policies, and avoid actions that may result in violations. This, in turn, mitigates legal and reputational risks for the organization.

7. **Employee Engagement and Empowerment:** Training and education programs empower employees by providing them with the knowledge and skills necessary to fulfill their compliance responsibilities. Engaged employees who understand their compliance obligations are more likely to take ownership of compliance efforts, actively participate in reporting and risk mitigation, and contribute to the overall success of the compliance program.

8. **Continuous Improvement and Adaptation:** Compliance training should be an ongoing process to keep up with evolving regulations, industry trends, and emerging compliance risks. Regular training and education

enable employees to stay updated and adapt to changes in the regulatory landscape. This ensures that compliance efforts remain effective and aligned with current requirements.

By investing in training and education programs, healthcare organizations can create a culture of compliance, enhance employee awareness and understanding of regulatory requirements, and mitigate compliance risks. It not only helps employees make informed decisions but also contributes to the overall success and integrity of the organization.

Designing Effective Compliance Training Programs

Designing effective compliance training programs requires careful planning and consideration (Figure 9.2). Here are key steps to follow in designing such programs:

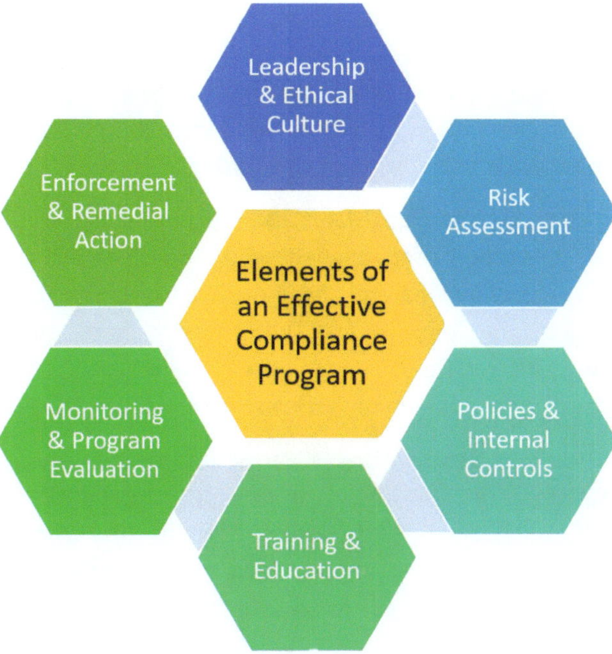

▼ **Figure 9.2:** Elements of an Effective Compliance Program

1. **Identify Training Objectives:** Define the specific objectives and desired outcomes of the training program. Determine the knowledge, skills, and behaviors that employees should acquire or improve through the training.

Align these objectives with the compliance goals and priorities of the organization.

2. **Conduct a Training Needs Assessment:** Assess the training needs of employees to identify knowledge gaps, areas of potential risk, and specific compliance challenges. Gather input from various stakeholders, including compliance professionals, managers, and employees themselves. This assessment helps tailor the training program to address the specific needs of the target audience.

3. **Define Training Content:** Based on the training objectives and needs assessment, determine the content areas that should be covered in the training program. Consider regulatory requirements, industry standards, internal policies, and any emerging compliance risks. Break down the content into modules or topics to ensure a structured and organized training curriculum.

4. **Select Appropriate Training Methods:** Choose the most suitable training methods and delivery formats based on the objectives, content, and target audience. Consider a combination of approaches, such as in-person sessions, e-learning modules, workshops, webinars, or simulations. The selected methods should engage participants, promote active learning, and provide opportunities for practice and reinforcement of key concepts.

5. **Develop Engaging Training Materials:** Create training materials that are engaging, interactive, and aligned with adult learning principles. Use a variety of instructional techniques, such as case studies, scenarios, group discussions, and quizzes, to enhance participant involvement and knowledge retention. Incorporate real-life examples and practical applications to make the training relevant to employees' daily work.

6. **Consider Different Learning Styles:** Recognize that individuals have different learning preferences and adapt the training program accordingly. Include visual aids, audio elements, hands-on activities, and written materials to cater to diverse learning styles. Providing training resources and materials in different formats allows participants to choose the method that best suits their preferences and needs.

7. **Include Role-Based Scenarios:** Tailor the training to different job roles within the organization. Develop role-specific scenarios and case studies that reflect the compliance challenges employees may encounter in their specific roles. This helps participants understand how compliance principles apply to their day-to-day tasks and reinforces the importance of compliance in their work.

8. **Provide Practical Guidance and Resources:** Offer practical guidance and resources that employees can refer to after the training. This may include compliance manuals, job aids, reference guides, and access to relevant policies and procedures. Ensure these resources are easily accessible and regularly updated to reflect changes in regulations or compliance requirements.

9. **Promote Engagement and Interaction:** Create opportunities for participant engagement and interaction throughout the training program. Encourage discussions, Q&A sessions, and group activities that allow participants to share experiences and learn from each other. This fosters a collaborative learning environment and enhances knowledge retention and application.

10. **Assess and Evaluate Training Effectiveness:** Establish methods to assess the effectiveness of the training program. Conduct pre- and post-training assessments to measure knowledge gained or behavior change. Gather feedback from participants to identify areas for improvement and assess the overall satisfaction with the training. Use the data collected to refine and enhance future training initiatives.

11. **Provide Ongoing Training and Refreshers:** Compliance training should not be a one-time event. Develop a plan for ongoing training and refreshers to keep employees updated with regulatory changes, emerging compliance risks, and new policies or procedures. This ensures that employees' knowledge remains current and their compliance skills are continuously reinforced.

By following these steps, healthcare organizations can design and implement effective compliance training programs that engage employees, enhance their understanding of compliance requirements, and promote a culture of compliance throughout the organization.

Engaging Employees in Compliance Initiatives

Engaging employees in compliance initiatives is crucial for creating a culture of compliance and ensuring the success of compliance programs. Here are some strategies to effectively engage employees in compliance:

1. **Communication and Transparency:** Foster open and transparent communication about compliance expectations, goals, and initiatives. Regularly communicate updates on regulatory changes, compliance policies, and any changes in compliance processes. Provide clarity on the importance

of compliance in achieving organizational objectives and emphasize the role that employees play in maintaining compliance.

2. **Leadership Commitment:** Ensure that leadership demonstrates a strong commitment to compliance. Leaders should lead by example, prioritize compliance in decision-making, and consistently communicate the organization's commitment to compliance. This commitment from leadership sets the tone for compliance throughout the organization and encourages employees to actively engage in compliance initiatives.

3. **Training and Education:** Provide comprehensive compliance training and education to employees at all levels. Offer training programs that are engaging, interactive, and relevant to their roles and responsibilities. Use real-life examples, case studies, and scenarios to make the training practical and relatable. Encourage employees to ask questions, seek clarification, and actively participate in the training process.

4. **Clear Policies and Procedures:** Develop clear and concise compliance policies and procedures that are easily accessible to employees. Ensure that employees understand the policies and procedures relevant to their roles and provide guidance on how to apply them in their daily work. Regularly communicate updates or changes to policies and procedures to keep employees informed.

5. **Employee Feedback and Input:** Encourage employees to provide feedback, suggestions, and input on compliance matters. Create channels for employees to report compliance concerns, ask questions, or seek guidance without fear of retaliation. Actively seek employee input during the development or revision of compliance policies, procedures, and training materials. Valuing and incorporating employee feedback fosters a sense of ownership and engagement in compliance initiatives.

6. **Recognition and Rewards:** Recognize and reward employees who demonstrate a commitment to compliance. Acknowledge and appreciate individuals or teams that go above and beyond in adhering to compliance standards or reporting compliance concerns. Publicly recognize compliance achievements to reinforce positive behaviors and promote a culture of compliance.

7. **Engagement through Committees and Champions:** Establish compliance committees or working groups consisting of employees from different departments. These committees can serve as ambassadors for compliance

initiatives and promote compliance awareness throughout the organization. Designate compliance champions within various departments who can act as advocates, provide guidance, and encourage their peers to actively engage in compliance efforts.

8. **Incorporate Compliance into Performance Evaluation:** Integrate compliance considerations into performance evaluations and goal-setting processes. Include compliance-related objectives or metrics as part of employees' performance evaluations, reinforcing the importance of compliance in their day-to-day work. Recognize and reward employees who consistently demonstrate a commitment to compliance in their performance evaluations.

9. **Regular Communication and Reinforcement:** Maintain regular communication about compliance initiatives through various channels such as newsletters, intranet portals, or team meetings. Reinforce compliance expectations through ongoing reminders, updates on regulatory changes, and sharing of best practices. Continuously emphasize the importance of compliance and its alignment with the organization's values and mission.

10. **Continuous Improvement and Learning:** Encourage a culture of continuous improvement and learning in compliance. Foster an environment where employees are encouraged to report compliance concerns, share lessons learned, and contribute to the enhancement of compliance processes. Promote ongoing learning through webinars, workshops, or other educational resources to keep employees updated on evolving compliance requirements.

By implementing these strategies, healthcare organizations can engage employees in compliance initiatives, foster a culture of compliance, and create a collective commitment to maintaining regulatory compliance throughout the organization.

Continuous Professional Development for Compliance Professionals

Continuous professional development is essential for compliance professionals to stay current with regulatory changes, industry trends, and best practices. Here are key aspects to consider for continuous professional development in compliance:

1. **Stay Informed about Regulatory Changes:** Regulatory landscapes are constantly evolving, and compliance professionals must proactively stay informed about new laws, regulations, and guidance relevant to their

industry. Regularly monitor regulatory updates, subscribe to industry newsletters, and follow reputable sources of information to stay abreast of changes that may impact compliance programs.

2. **Participate in Industry Events and Conferences:** Attend conferences, seminars, and workshops related to compliance and regulatory affairs. These events provide opportunities to learn from industry experts, gain insights into emerging compliance trends, and network with peers. Look for events that offer sessions specific to compliance challenges and provide continuing education credits, where applicable.

3. **Professional Associations and Networks:** Join professional associations and networks dedicated to compliance and regulatory affairs. These organizations offer access to resources, research, training, and networking opportunities with other compliance professionals. Engage in online discussion forums, attend webinars, and contribute to the knowledge-sharing within these communities.

4. **Certifications and Credentials:** Pursue relevant certifications and credentials in compliance. Certifications, such as Certified Compliance and Ethics Professional (CCEP), Certified Regulatory Compliance Manager (CRCM), or Certified in Healthcare Compliance (CHC), demonstrate expertise and commitment to the compliance profession. These certifications often require ongoing education to maintain and renew the credential.

5. **Continuing Education Programs:** Engage in continuing education programs focused on compliance. Many institutions offer specialized courses or executive education programs that cover various aspects of compliance, including regulatory requirements, risk management, ethics, and leadership. These programs can enhance knowledge and skills while providing opportunities for networking and learning from industry experts.

6. **Internal Training and Mentorship:** Take advantage of internal training opportunities provided by your organization. Attend internal compliance workshops, seminars, or webinars to enhance your knowledge of organizational policies, procedures, and specific compliance challenges. Seek mentorship from experienced compliance professionals within your organization to learn from their expertise and gain practical insights.

7. **Reading and Research:** Continuously invest time in reading and researching compliance-related topics. Stay updated with compliance literature, industry publications, regulatory guidance, and relevant academic research.

Regularly review professional journals, articles, and whitepapers to deepen your understanding of compliance concepts and gain insights into emerging practices.

8. **Cross-Functional Collaboration:** Collaborate with professionals from other departments within your organization, such as legal, risk management, and internal audit. Participate in cross-functional meetings or projects to broaden your understanding of different perspectives and enhance your knowledge of related disciplines. This collaboration helps build a holistic understanding of compliance and fosters a multidisciplinary approach to risk management.

9. **Continuous Learning Culture:** Embrace a culture of continuous learning and encourage your compliance team and colleagues to prioritize professional development. Share relevant articles, resources, and training opportunities with your team. Foster a supportive environment where knowledge-sharing and learning from each other's experiences are valued.

10. **Self-Assessment and Development Plans:** Regularly assess your own knowledge, skills, and areas for growth. Identify areas where you would benefit from additional training or development. Create a personal development plan that outlines specific goals, actions, and timelines for enhancing your expertise in those areas. Regularly review and update your development plan to ensure progress and growth.

Continuous professional development is vital for compliance professionals to adapt to regulatory changes, develop new skills, and maintain the highest level of expertise in their field. By actively engaging in ongoing learning, compliance professionals can ensure their effectiveness in navigating the complex compliance landscape and contribute to the success of their organizations' compliance programs.

Chapter 10

Case Studies and Best Practices

This chapter delves into real-world case studies and best practices in regulatory compliance within the healthcare industry. Drawing from actual scenarios and success stories, this chapter provides valuable insights and practical examples of how organizations have navigated compliance challenges and implemented effective compliance programs. Chapter 10 offers readers valuable insights into the practical application of regulatory compliance in the healthcare industry. It helps compliance professionals understand the complexities of compliance, learn from the experiences of others, and implement effective strategies and approaches within their own organizations. The chapter serves as a guide for achieving regulatory compliance excellence and maintaining a culture of integrity and ethical conduct in healthcare organizations.

Real-world Case Studies Highlighting Compliance Challenges and their Resolutions

Case Study 1: Healthcare Data Breach Response

Challenge: A healthcare organization experienced a data breach that exposed sensitive patient information, including medical records and personally identifiable information (PII). The breach raised significant concerns regarding patient privacy and compliance with healthcare privacy regulations.

Resolution: The organization responded to the breach by promptly initiating an incident response plan. They engaged a specialized cybersecurity firm to conduct a forensic investigation to determine the extent of the breach, identify vulnerabilities, and mitigate further risks. The organization also notified affected individuals and implemented measures to secure the compromised data. They worked closely with regulatory authorities, such as the Office for Civil Rights (OCR) in the United States, to ensure compliance with breach notification requirements. As a result, the organization enhanced their data security measures, implemented encryption protocols, and provided additional training to employees on data privacy and security.

Lessons Learned: This case study emphasizes the importance of having a robust incident response plan in place to effectively handle data breaches. Prompt action, collaboration with cybersecurity experts, and clear communication with affected individuals and regulatory authorities are crucial. Organizations should continuously review and enhance their data security measures to prevent future breaches and ensure compliance with privacy regulations.

Case Study 2: Fraudulent Billing Scheme Detection

Challenge: A healthcare organization discovered a fraudulent billing scheme where a group of employees manipulated billing codes and submitted false claims for services that were not provided. The scheme resulted in significant financial losses for the organization and raised concerns about compliance with billing and coding regulations.

Resolution: The organization conducted an internal investigation, working closely with their compliance department and auditors. They identified the individuals involved in the fraudulent scheme and terminated their employment. The organization implemented additional controls and audits to prevent similar incidents in the future. They also enhanced their compliance training programs, specifically focusing on educating employees about proper billing and coding practices, as well as the consequences of fraudulent activities. The organization proactively cooperated with relevant regulatory agencies during the investigation and implemented recommended changes to their billing processes to ensure compliance.

Lessons Learned: This case study underscores the importance of strong internal controls and regular audits to detect and prevent fraudulent activities. Effective compliance training, clear policies, and strict enforcement of ethical standards are crucial to ensure employees understand their obligations and the potential consequences of non-compliance. Cooperation with regulatory agencies and implementing their recommendations demonstrates a commitment to compliance and rebuilding trust within the organization.

Case Study 3: Research Ethics and Human Subjects Protection

Challenge: A healthcare organization conducting clinical trials faced an ethical dilemma regarding the informed consent process for participants. The organization realized that some participants did not fully comprehend the risks and benefits of participating in the trial, potentially compromising the ethical principles of informed consent.

Resolution: The organization reviewed and revised their informed consent procedures to ensure they met the highest ethical standards. They sought guidance from their Institutional Review Board (IRB) and engaged with research ethics experts to develop clearer, more comprehensive informed consent documents. They also enhanced the training and education provided to researchers and staff involved in clinical trials to emphasize the importance of informed consent and ethical conduct in research. The organization implemented a robust monitoring and auditing process to ensure ongoing compliance with human subjects protection regulations.

Lessons Learned: This case study highlights the critical role of research ethics and the need for organizations to continuously evaluate and enhance their processes related to informed consent. Collaborating with experts, such as IRBs, helps ensure adherence to ethical guidelines. Training and education programs for researchers and staff should emphasize the significance of informed consent and ethical conduct, fostering a culture of research integrity and patient protection.

These case studies illustrate real-world compliance challenges faced by healthcare organizations and the actions taken to address them. By examining these scenarios, compliance professionals can gain insights into effective strategies for resolving compliance issues and implementing preventive measures to avoid similar challenges in the future.

Best Practices for Achieving and Maintaining Regulatory Compliance

Achieving and maintaining regulatory compliance in the healthcare industry requires a systematic approach and adherence to best practices. Here are key best practices to consider:

1. **Develop a Compliance Program:** Establish a comprehensive compliance program that includes policies, procedures, and processes to address

regulatory requirements. Designate a compliance officer or team responsible for overseeing the program and ensuring its effectiveness.

2. **Stay Abreast of Regulatory Changes:** Regularly monitor and stay informed about changes in regulations, laws, and guidelines that affect your organization. This includes following updates from regulatory bodies and participating in industry forums and associations.

3. **Conduct Regular Risk Assessments:** Perform periodic risk assessments to identify potential compliance risks and vulnerabilities within your organization. Prioritize risks based on their likelihood and potential impact. Use the assessment results to develop risk management strategies and action plans.

4. **Educate and Train Employees:** Provide comprehensive compliance training to all employees at various levels of the organization. Training should cover regulatory requirements, internal policies, and ethical considerations. Ensure employees understand their compliance responsibilities and are equipped to make informed decisions.

5. **Implement Internal Controls:** Establish internal controls to mitigate compliance risks and ensure adherence to regulatory requirements. Internal controls may include segregation of duties, regular audits, monitoring processes, and implementing technology solutions to automate compliance monitoring.

6. **Promote a Culture of Compliance:** Foster a culture where compliance is prioritized and embedded in everyday operations. Leadership should set a positive example, encourage open communication, and recognize and reward ethical behavior. Encourage employees to report concerns and create a non-retaliatory environment for whistleblowing.

7. **Monitor and Audit Compliance:** Regularly monitor and audit compliance activities to ensure ongoing adherence to regulatory requirements. Conduct internal audits, self-assessments, and periodic reviews of compliance processes. Address identified issues promptly and implement corrective actions.

8. **Establish Clear Policies and Procedures:** Develop clear and accessible policies and procedures that outline compliance expectations, processes, and guidelines. Ensure policies are regularly reviewed, updated, and communicated to employees.

9. **Maintain Documentation and Record Keeping:** Keep thorough and organized documentation of compliance activities, including policies, procedures, training records, audit reports, and incident responses. Proper documentation serves as evidence of compliance efforts and facilitates external audits or regulatory inspections.

10. **Engage in External Collaboration:** Collaborate with industry associations, peers, and external experts to stay informed about emerging best practices and regulatory trends. Participate in industry conferences, forums, and networking events to share knowledge and learn from others' experiences.

11. **Respond to Non-Compliance:** Establish a process for addressing and responding to instances of non-compliance. Promptly investigate reported concerns, implement corrective actions, and take appropriate disciplinary measures when necessary. Foster a culture of accountability and continuous improvement.

12. **Regularly Review and Update Compliance Program:** Continuously evaluate and update your compliance program to reflect changes in regulations, industry standards, and organizational needs. Regularly assess the effectiveness of compliance initiatives and make necessary improvements based on lessons learned.

By adopting these best practices, healthcare organizations can enhance their regulatory compliance efforts, reduce compliance risks, and ensure the delivery of safe and high-quality care to patients while maintaining the trust of stakeholders and regulatory bodies.

Lessons Learned from Successful Compliance Programs

Lessons learned from successful compliance programs provide valuable insights into effective strategies and approaches for achieving and maintaining regulatory compliance. Here are some key lessons learned:

1. **Leadership Commitment and Tone from the Top:** Successful compliance programs require strong leadership commitment and a clear tone from the top. When leaders prioritize compliance, set a positive example, and communicate the importance of compliance throughout the organization, it creates a culture where compliance is valued and embedded in day-to-day operations.

2. **Comprehensive Risk Assessment:** Conducting thorough risk assessments is critical for identifying compliance risks specific to the organization. Successful compliance programs regularly assess internal and external risks, including regulatory changes, operational vulnerabilities, and emerging industry risks. This allows organizations to prioritize their compliance efforts and allocate resources effectively.

3. **Tailored Policies and Procedures:** Developing clear and concise compliance policies and procedures is essential. These should be tailored to the organization's specific operations, industry regulations, and compliance risks. Successful compliance programs ensure that policies and procedures are accessible, regularly updated, and communicated effectively to all employees.

4. **Education and Training:** Continuous education and training programs are essential for promoting compliance awareness and building employees' knowledge and skills. Successful compliance programs offer comprehensive training on regulatory requirements, ethical conduct, and reporting obligations. Training should be interactive, engaging, and customized to different employee roles and responsibilities.

5. **Effective Communication and Reporting Channels:** Open and effective communication channels are vital for encouraging employees to report compliance concerns and seek guidance. Successful compliance programs establish confidential reporting mechanisms, such as anonymous hotlines or online portals, to encourage employees to report potential violations. Clear communication ensures employees understand reporting procedures and are confident in raising compliance issues.

6. **Monitoring, Auditing, and Internal Controls:** Implementing robust monitoring and auditing processes is crucial for detecting and addressing compliance violations. Successful compliance programs conduct regular audits, monitor key compliance metrics, and implement internal controls to mitigate risks. Regular monitoring allows organizations to proactively identify compliance gaps, promptly address issues, and ensure ongoing compliance.

7. **Continuous Improvement and Adaptation:** Compliance programs should continually evolve to address emerging risks and changes in regulations. Successful programs embrace a culture of continuous improvement, regularly review and enhance policies and procedures, and incorporate lessons learned from internal and external audits or incidents. Organizations that adapt to

evolving compliance requirements are better equipped to maintain regulatory compliance.

8. **Collaboration and Stakeholder Engagement:** Successful compliance programs foster collaboration and engagement among various stakeholders, including employees, managers, legal counsel, auditors, and regulators. Engaging stakeholders enhances compliance effectiveness, facilitates timely resolution of compliance issues, and demonstrates a commitment to ethical conduct and regulatory compliance.

9. **Documented Compliance Efforts:** Documenting compliance efforts, including policies, procedures, training materials, and audit reports, is crucial for demonstrating a proactive compliance program. Successful programs maintain accurate and up-to-date records of compliance activities, including risk assessments, training records, and incident investigations. Documentation provides evidence of compliance efforts and helps in responding to audits or regulatory inquiries.

10. **Regular Evaluation and External Benchmarking:** Successful compliance programs regularly evaluate their effectiveness and benchmark against industry best practices. Conducting periodic assessments allows organizations to identify areas for improvement, address compliance gaps, and compare their compliance practices with industry peers. External benchmarking provides valuable insights and helps organizations stay ahead in the evolving regulatory landscape.

By incorporating these lessons learned into compliance programs, healthcare organizations can enhance their regulatory compliance efforts, mitigate risks, and foster a culture of integrity and ethical conduct.

Innovations and Emerging Practices in Healthcare Compliance

Innovations and emerging practices in healthcare compliance are transforming the way organizations manage compliance risks and meet regulatory requirements. Here are some key innovations and practices that are shaping healthcare compliance:

1. **Data Analytics and Artificial Intelligence (AI):** Healthcare organizations are leveraging data analytics and AI technologies to enhance compliance monitoring, risk assessment, and detection of potential compliance issues.

These technologies can analyze large volumes of data to identify patterns, anomalies, and potential compliance violations, allowing organizations to take proactive measures to address risks and ensure compliance.

2. **Robotic Process Automation (RPA):** RPA is being used to automate repetitive and manual compliance tasks, such as data entry, record keeping, and report generation. By automating these processes, organizations can improve efficiency, accuracy, and consistency in compliance-related activities, while freeing up resources to focus on more strategic compliance initiatives.

3. **Blockchain Technology:** Blockchain technology offers potential applications in healthcare compliance, particularly in areas such as data security, privacy, and supply chain management. Blockchain can provide secure, transparent, and immutable record-keeping, ensuring the integrity and traceability of compliance-related transactions and data.

4. **Telehealth Compliance:** The rapid growth of telehealth services has introduced unique compliance considerations. Healthcare organizations must navigate regulatory requirements related to telehealth, such as licensure, privacy, and reimbursement. Compliance programs are adapting to incorporate specific telehealth compliance protocols to ensure that patient privacy is protected, informed consent is obtained, and telehealth services meet regulatory standards.

5. **Privacy by Design:** Privacy by Design is an approach that embeds privacy and data protection principles into the design of systems, processes, and technologies. Healthcare organizations are increasingly adopting Privacy by Design practices to proactively address privacy and data protection requirements and ensure compliance from the outset.

6. **Vendor and Third-Party Risk Management:** Healthcare organizations are focusing on managing compliance risks associated with vendors and third-party relationships. This includes implementing robust vendor due diligence processes, conducting regular assessments of vendor compliance, and establishing contractual provisions that require compliance with applicable regulations and standards.

7. **Compliance Training through Technology:** Technology-enabled training solutions, such as e-learning platforms, virtual reality (VR), and mobile applications, are being utilized to deliver engaging and interactive compliance training programs. These platforms provide flexibility, scalability, and real-time tracking of training completion and effectiveness.

8. **Proactive Compliance Monitoring and Auditing:** Instead of relying solely on retrospective audits, organizations are adopting real-time monitoring and auditing capabilities to detect and address compliance issues in a timely manner. This includes leveraging data analytics, AI, and automation to continuously monitor compliance metrics, conduct risk assessments, and identify potential compliance violations.

9. **Compliance Gamification:** Gamification techniques, such as incorporating game elements and rewards into compliance training and reporting, are being used to engage employees and encourage active participation in compliance initiatives. Gamification enhances the learning experience, increases retention, and fosters a positive compliance culture.

10. **Collaborative Compliance Platforms:** Healthcare organizations are exploring collaborative compliance platforms that facilitate communication, information sharing, and collaboration among compliance professionals. These platforms enable organizations to share best practices, access compliance resources, and collaborate on addressing common compliance challenges.

By embracing these innovations and emerging practices, healthcare organizations can enhance their compliance programs, improve efficiency, and effectively manage compliance risks in an ever-changing regulatory landscape. It is important for organizations to stay abreast of these developments and carefully assess their applicability and potential impact on their specific compliance needs.

Compliance in Health Information Technology

Compliance in health information technology (HIT) refers to the adherence to regulatory requirements, standards, and best practices in the design, implementation, and use of technology systems that store, manage, and exchange health information. Compliance in HIT is crucial for protecting patient privacy, ensuring data security, promoting interoperability, and facilitating the effective and safe use of health IT systems. Here are key aspects of compliance in health information technology:

1. **Regulatory Framework:** Compliance in HIT is governed by various regulations, including the Health Insurance Portability and Accountability Act (HIPAA), the Health Information Technology for Economic and Clinical Health (HITECH) Act, and the 21st Century Cures Act. These regulations set requirements for the protection of patient health information, electronic health record (EHR) systems, and the secure exchange of health data.

2. **Privacy and Security:** Compliance in HIT involves implementing privacy and security measures to protect electronic protected health information (ePHI) from unauthorized access, use, or disclosure. This includes conducting risk assessments, implementing administrative, physical, and technical safeguards, training employees on privacy and security policies, and responding to breaches in accordance with breach notification requirements.

3. **Interoperability and Data Exchange:** Compliance in HIT also encompasses ensuring interoperability and seamless data exchange between different health IT systems and entities. This involves complying with interoperability standards and protocols, such as Fast Healthcare Interoperability Resources (FHIR), and implementing secure health information exchange (HIE) mechanisms to facilitate the exchange of patient health information.

4. **Health IT Governance:** Compliance in HIT requires the establishment of effective governance structures and compliance programs. This includes

developing HIT policies and procedures, conducting regular audits and assessments to identify compliance gaps, providing training to employees on HIT compliance requirements, and implementing ongoing monitoring and corrective actions to ensure continued compliance.

5. **Cybersecurity:** Compliance in HIT includes implementing robust cybersecurity measures to protect health IT systems from cyber threats. This involves implementing firewalls, intrusion detection systems, encryption, and access controls, as well as regularly monitoring and responding to security incidents. Compliance with cybersecurity frameworks and standards, such as the National Institute of Standards and Technology (NIST) Cybersecurity Framework, is also essential.

6. **Vendor Management:** Compliance in HIT extends to managing the compliance of HIT vendors and third-party service providers. This includes conducting due diligence assessments, ensuring contracts include appropriate compliance requirements, and regularly monitoring vendor compliance with relevant regulations and standards.

7. **Emerging Technologies:** Compliance in HIT also encompasses considering the compliance implications of emerging technologies, such as artificial intelligence (AI), machine learning, blockchain, and Internet of Things (IoT), as they are integrated into health IT systems. Understanding the regulatory requirements and ethical considerations associated with these technologies is essential for ensuring compliance.

Compliance in health information technology is an ongoing effort that requires collaboration among healthcare organizations, HIT vendors, regulators, and other stakeholders. It involves staying abreast of regulatory changes, adopting best practices, and continually assessing and improving HIT systems to ensure they meet compliance requirements while enabling the delivery of high-quality and secure healthcare services.

Regulatory Requirements for Health Information Technology (HIT) Systems

Regulatory requirements for health information technology (HIT) systems are designed to protect the privacy, security, and interoperability of health information while promoting the effective use of technology in healthcare. Here are some key regulatory requirements for HIT systems:

1. **Health Insurance Portability and Accountability Act (HIPAA):** HIPAA establishes the standards for the privacy and security of protected health information (PHI). Covered entities, such as healthcare providers, health plans, and healthcare clearinghouses, must comply with HIPAA's Privacy Rule and Security Rule when handling PHI. The Privacy Rule sets requirements for the use and disclosure of PHI, while the Security Rule establishes safeguards to protect electronic PHI (ePHI).

2. **Health Information Technology for Economic and Clinical Health (HITECH) Act:** The HITECH Act complements HIPAA by expanding the privacy and security provisions and strengthening the enforcement of HIPAA requirements. It also promotes the adoption of electronic health records (EHRs) and the secure exchange of health information through health information exchange (HIE) networks.

3. **21st Century Cures Act:** The 21st Century Cures Act focuses on advancing healthcare innovation, including health IT. It aims to improve interoperability and patient access to health information. The act mandates that certified EHR technology supports the seamless exchange of health information and prohibits information blocking by healthcare providers, health IT developers, and health information networks.

4. **Centers for Medicare and Medicaid Services (CMS) Regulations:** CMS regulations govern HIT systems used by healthcare providers participating in the Medicare and Medicaid programs. These regulations include the Electronic Health Record (EHR) Incentive Programs, which provide financial incentives to eligible professionals and hospitals that adopt and meaningfully use certified EHR technology.

5. **Food and Drug Administration (FDA) Regulations:** The FDA regulates HIT systems that meet the definition of medical devices. Certain HIT systems, such as medical device software and mobile medical applications, may require FDA clearance or approval before they can be marketed and used in patient care.

6. **Office of the National Coordinator for Health Information Technology (ONC) Certification Program:** The ONC Certification Program establishes criteria and standards for the certification of EHR technology. It ensures that EHR systems meet specific functionality, interoperability, and security requirements to support the meaningful use of health information and participate in incentive programs.

7. **State-specific Laws and Regulations:** In addition to federal regulations, individual states may have their own laws and regulations that govern HIT systems. These state laws may address additional privacy and security requirements, licensing requirements, or specific provisions related to health information exchange within the state.

Compliance with these regulatory requirements is essential for healthcare organizations and HIT vendors to protect patient privacy, ensure data security, promote interoperability, and meet eligibility criteria for incentive programs. It is important to stay updated with changes to these regulations and ensure that HIT systems and processes are designed, implemented, and maintained in accordance with the applicable requirements.

Electronic Health Records (EHR) Interoperability and Data Exchange

Electronic health records (EHR) interoperability and data exchange refer to the ability of different EHR systems and healthcare organizations to securely and seamlessly share patient health information. Interoperability and data exchange are crucial for improving care coordination, enhancing patient safety, and enabling the efficient and effective exchange of health information between healthcare providers. Here are key aspects of EHR interoperability and data exchange:

1. **Standards and Protocols:** Interoperability relies on the use of standardized data formats, coding systems, and communication protocols to ensure that EHR systems can understand and exchange health information effectively. Standards, such as the HL7 (Health Level Seven) and the Fast Healthcare Interoperability Resources (FHIR), provide a common language and structure for health data exchange.

2. **Health Information Exchange (HIE) Networks:** HIE networks facilitate the secure exchange of health information between different healthcare organizations, including hospitals, clinics, laboratories, and pharmacies. These networks serve as intermediaries that enable the transmission of health data while adhering to privacy and security requirements.

3. **Direct Messaging:** Direct messaging is a secure email-like system that allows healthcare providers to exchange patient health information directly with other authorized healthcare providers. It enables point-to-point communication and is commonly used for sending referrals, discharge summaries, and lab results.

4. **Query-Based Exchange:** Query-based exchange enables healthcare providers to electronically search and retrieve patient health information from external EHR systems or health information exchanges. This method allows authorized providers to access specific patient data when needed, such as during emergency situations or when treating patients with complex medical histories.

5. **Consent and Privacy Controls:** EHR interoperability and data exchange require appropriate consent and privacy controls to ensure that patient privacy is protected. Patients have the right to control how their health information is shared, and systems should support consent management and secure data access controls to comply with privacy regulations, such as HIPAA.

6. **Patient Access to Health Information:** EHR interoperability promotes patient engagement by enabling individuals to access their health information electronically. Patients can view, download, and transmit their health records, empowering them to actively participate in their care and share information with other healthcare providers or third-party applications.

7. **Interoperability Testing and Certification:** EHR systems can undergo interoperability testing and certification programs to ensure their compliance with interoperability standards and protocols. These programs validate that EHR systems can effectively exchange data with other systems and participate in health information exchange initiatives.

8. **Nationwide Interoperability Initiatives:** Governments and healthcare organizations worldwide are promoting nationwide interoperability initiatives to establish a seamless flow of health information across organizations and regions. These initiatives aim to overcome technical, organizational, and policy barriers to achieve comprehensive EHR interoperability and data exchange.

Achieving EHR interoperability and data exchange requires collaboration among healthcare organizations, EHR vendors, government entities, and standards development organizations. It involves aligning technical infrastructure, implementing data governance policies, and ensuring compliance with privacy and security regulations. The goal is to enable healthcare providers to access complete and accurate patient information at the point of care, leading to improved care coordination, clinical decision-making, and patient outcomes.

Health Information Privacy and Security Considerations in HIT

Health information privacy and security considerations are critical in health information technology (HIT) to protect the confidentiality, integrity, and availability of patient health information. Safeguarding sensitive health data is essential to maintain patient trust, comply with regulatory requirements, and prevent unauthorized access or breaches. Here are key health information privacy and security considerations in HIT:

1. **HIPAA Compliance:** Compliance with the Health Insurance Portability and Accountability Act (HIPAA) is paramount. Covered entities and their business associates must adhere to HIPAA's Privacy Rule and Security Rule to protect the privacy and security of protected health information (PHI) and electronic protected health information (ePHI). This includes implementing safeguards, conducting risk assessments, and ensuring appropriate administrative, physical, and technical safeguards are in place.

2. **Access Controls:** Implementing strong access controls is crucial to prevent unauthorized access to patient health information. This involves authentication mechanisms such as unique usernames and passwords, multi-factor authentication, and role-based access controls (RBAC) to ensure that only authorized individuals can access and view specific patient data.

3. **Encryption:** Encryption plays a vital role in protecting health information during transmission and storage. Implementing encryption technologies, such as Secure Sockets Layer (SSL) or Transport Layer Security (TLS) protocols, ensures that data is encrypted when transmitted over networks. Encryption of data at rest, such as using encryption keys to protect stored health information, adds an additional layer of security.

4. **Auditing and Monitoring:** Robust auditing and monitoring mechanisms are necessary to detect and respond to potential security incidents or unauthorized access. Implementing audit trails, logs, and intrusion detection systems allows organizations to track and monitor user activities, identify anomalies or suspicious behavior, and investigate any breaches or security breaches promptly.

5. **Data Backup and Disaster Recovery:** Health information systems should have comprehensive data backup and disaster recovery plans in place to ensure the availability and integrity of patient data in the event of system

failures, natural disasters, or other emergencies. Regularly backing up data and testing recovery processes help mitigate risks and ensure data can be restored promptly.

6. **Training and Awareness:** Providing comprehensive privacy and security training to employees is essential. Staff members should be educated on the importance of safeguarding patient information, recognizing potential security threats, and understanding their roles and responsibilities in protecting health information. Ongoing awareness programs help reinforce good security practices and promote a culture of privacy and security within the organization.

7. **Business Associate Agreements:** Health information shared with third-party vendors or business associates should be protected through robust business associate agreements (BAAs). These agreements outline the responsibilities of the business associates in safeguarding PHI or ePHI and ensure compliance with privacy and security requirements.

8. **Incident Response and Breach Notification:** Establishing incident response plans and breach notification protocols is crucial to respond swiftly and appropriately to security incidents or breaches. Organizations should have procedures in place to assess and mitigate the impact of breaches, notify affected individuals and regulatory authorities, and take necessary steps to prevent future incidents.

9. **Vendor Security Assessments:** Conducting thorough security assessments of HIT vendors is essential when selecting and engaging with external vendors or utilizing cloud-based services. Organizations should evaluate the security measures implemented by vendors, including data encryption, access controls, vulnerability management, and compliance with industry security standards.

10. **Regulatory Compliance Audits:** Regular internal and external audits help ensure ongoing compliance with privacy and security regulations. Conducting internal audits and engaging independent third-party auditors can identify gaps or weaknesses in security practices, provide recommendations for improvement, and demonstrate a commitment to maintaining a robust privacy and security posture.

By addressing these health information privacy and security considerations, healthcare organizations can protect patient data, meet regulatory requirements, and maintain the confidentiality and integrity of health information in HIT systems.

Implementing comprehensive privacy and security measures creates a foundation of trust and confidence among patients, healthcare providers, and other stakeholders in the secure and responsible handling of sensitive health information.

Compliance Challenges in Implementing and Maintaining HIT Systems

Implementing and maintaining health information technology (HIT) systems comes with several compliance challenges that organizations must navigate. These challenges arise from the complexity of healthcare regulations, evolving technology landscape, and the need to balance usability with security and privacy (Figure 11.1). Here are some common compliance challenges in implementing and maintaining HIT systems:

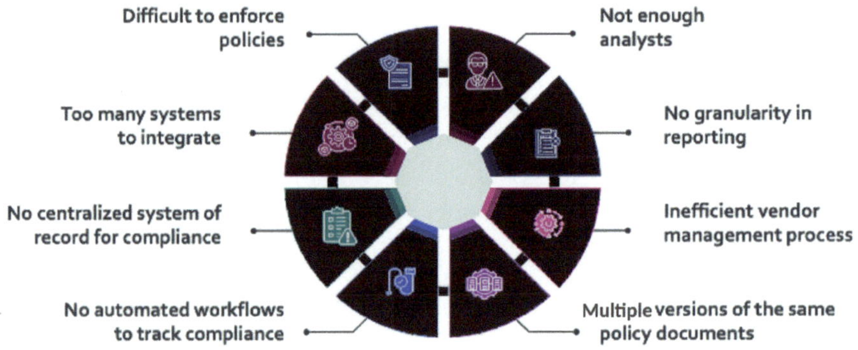

▼ **Figure 11.1:** Challenges in Compliance

1. **Regulatory Compliance:** HIT systems must comply with various regulations, such as HIPAA, HITECH Act, and state-specific laws. Ensuring adherence to these regulations, including privacy, security, and data breach notification requirements, can be complex, requiring ongoing monitoring, policy updates, and staff training to maintain compliance.

2. **Interoperability and Data Exchange:** Achieving seamless interoperability and data exchange between different EHR systems and healthcare organizations can be challenging. Technical, organizational, and policy barriers can hinder the sharing of health information, making it difficult to achieve true data interoperability and exchange while ensuring privacy and security.

3. **Data Privacy and Security:** Protecting patient privacy and ensuring data security is a critical challenge. HIT systems handle sensitive patient health information, and organizations must implement robust privacy and security measures, such as access controls, encryption, and data breach response protocols, to safeguard this information from unauthorized access or breaches.

4. **Vendor Management:** Working with HIT vendors introduces compliance challenges, especially when it comes to assessing and ensuring the compliance of vendor products or services. Organizations must carefully evaluate vendor contracts, conduct due diligence assessments, and monitor vendors' compliance with privacy, security, and regulatory requirements.

5. **User Training and Awareness:** User training and awareness are crucial for compliance, but they can be challenging to implement effectively. Training staff on the proper use of HIT systems, privacy practices, security protocols, and compliance requirements is essential for maintaining a culture of compliance. Regular training updates and ongoing reinforcement are necessary due to staff turnover and evolving regulations.

6. **Usability and Workflow Integration:** Balancing usability and workflow integration with compliance requirements can be a challenge. HIT systems must be user-friendly, efficient, and seamlessly integrate into existing healthcare workflows. However, compliance considerations, such as capturing and documenting required data elements, can sometimes disrupt clinical workflows and lead to user dissatisfaction.

7. **Data Integrity and Accuracy:** Maintaining data integrity and accuracy is crucial for compliance. HIT systems must capture, store, and transmit data accurately, ensuring that information is not lost, altered, or misrepresented. Organizations need proper data governance processes, validation procedures, and data quality checks to ensure compliance with data integrity standards.

8. **Audit Readiness and Documentation:** Organizations must be prepared for audits and be able to provide documentation and evidence of compliance with regulations and standards. Maintaining proper documentation, conducting internal audits, and implementing effective controls and processes are essential for audit readiness and compliance validation.

9. **Emerging Technologies and Standards:** The rapid pace of technological advancements, such as AI, IoT, and cloud computing, introduces new

compliance challenges. Organizations must stay updated on emerging technologies, assess their compliance implications, and adapt their systems and processes to meet evolving standards and regulatory requirements.

10. **Legacy Systems and Data Migration:** Replacing or upgrading legacy systems and migrating data to new HIT systems can be complex and pose compliance challenges. Organizations must ensure that data migration processes maintain data integrity, security, and compliance during the transition from legacy systems to newer technologies.

Navigating these compliance challenges requires a proactive approach, collaboration between IT and compliance teams, continuous monitoring of regulatory changes, and a commitment to ongoing training and education. Organizations must also engage with industry associations, regulatory bodies, and HIT vendors to stay informed about best practices and compliance solutions specific to HIT systems.

Chapter 12

Compliance in Health Insurance and Payer Relations

Compliance in health insurance and payer relations refers to the adherence to regulatory requirements, industry standards, and contractual obligations in the context of health insurance operations and interactions with insurance payers. Health insurance organizations, including insurance companies, managed care organizations, and third-party administrators, must comply with various regulations and ensure ethical and transparent practices in their relationships with insurance payers. Here are key aspects of compliance in health insurance and payer relations:

1. **Regulatory Compliance:** Health insurance organizations must comply with federal and state regulations that govern the insurance industry, such as the Affordable Care Act (ACA), the Employee Retirement Income Security Act (ERISA), and state insurance laws. Compliance includes licensing requirements, financial solvency regulations, rate filing obligations, claims processing standards, and consumer protection provisions.

2. **Contractual Obligations:** Health insurance organizations enter into contractual agreements with insurance payers, such as employer groups or government programs. Compliance in payer relations involves fulfilling contractual obligations, including network participation agreements, claims processing, reimbursement rates, utilization management requirements, and reporting obligations.

3. **Provider Network Compliance:** Health insurance organizations must maintain compliant provider networks by ensuring network adequacy, credentialing and re-credentialing providers, and monitoring network quality and performance. Compliance includes following state and federal regulations related to network adequacy standards, timely access to care, and provider reimbursement practices.

4. **Claims Processing and Adjudication:** Compliance in claims processing and adjudication involves accurate and timely handling of claims submitted by

healthcare providers. Health insurance organizations must adhere to claims submission guidelines, claims coding and documentation requirements (such as using appropriate CPT and ICD codes), and regulatory requirements for claim payment, appeals, and grievances.

5. **Fraud and Abuse Prevention:** Health insurance organizations have a responsibility to prevent fraud, waste, and abuse in the insurance system. Compliance efforts include implementing anti-fraud programs, conducting fraud investigations, monitoring provider billing practices, and participating in fraud reporting and prevention initiatives.

6. **Consumer Protection and Privacy:** Compliance in health insurance and payer relations also encompasses protecting consumer rights and privacy. Health insurance organizations must comply with regulations such as HIPAA, which governs the privacy and security of protected health information (PHI). Compliance includes obtaining and managing informed consent, providing access to health information, and implementing security safeguards to protect sensitive consumer data.

7. **Quality Improvement Initiatives:** Health insurance organizations may be required to participate in quality improvement initiatives, such as the Healthcare Effectiveness Data and Information Set (HEDIS), to measure and improve healthcare quality and outcomes. Compliance includes data reporting, performance measurement, and participation in quality improvement activities.

8. **Government Programs Compliance:** Health insurance organizations that participate in government-funded programs, such as Medicare and Medicaid, must comply with specific program requirements, including program integrity standards, claims submission guidelines, and compliance with program rules and regulations.

9. **Internal Audits and Monitoring:** Health insurance organizations should conduct internal audits and monitoring activities to assess compliance with regulatory requirements, contractual obligations, and internal policies. Compliance audits help identify areas of non-compliance, implement corrective actions, and ensure ongoing compliance.

10. **Collaboration with Payers:** Collaboration between health insurance organizations and insurance payers is essential for compliance. Engaging in open communication, sharing information on policy changes, negotiating contracts, and participating in payer meetings or committees help foster compliance and ensure alignment with payer requirements.

Compliance in health insurance and payer relations requires a comprehensive understanding of regulatory requirements, contractual obligations, and ethical practices. It involves close collaboration with internal departments, providers, and insurance payers to establish and maintain compliant operations and relationships. Regular monitoring, staff training, and proactive compliance measures are essential to meet regulatory expectations and promote ethical and transparent interactions in the health insurance industry.

Overview of Health Insurance Regulations (ACA, ERISA)

Health insurance regulations play a crucial role in governing the health insurance industry, ensuring consumer protection, promoting access to affordable coverage, and establishing standards for insurance providers (Table 12.1). Here's an overview of two key health insurance regulations:

▼ **Table 12.1:** Health Insurance Regulations

Regulation	Description
Affordable Care Act (ACA)	Legislation that regulates health insurance coverage, including requirements for essential health benefits and cost-sharing limits.
Employee Retirement Income Security Act (ERISA)	Federal law that sets standards for employee benefit plans offered by private employers, including health insurance.

1. **Affordable Care Act (ACA):** The Affordable Care Act, also known as Obamacare, was enacted in 2010 with the goal of expanding access to affordable health insurance and improving the quality and affordability of healthcare in the United States. Key provisions of the ACA include:

   • **Individual Mandate:** The ACA required most individuals to have health insurance coverage or pay a penalty. However, the individual mandate penalty was reduced to $0 starting from 2019.

   • **Marketplace Exchanges:** The ACA established Health Insurance Marketplaces (also called Exchanges) where individuals and small businesses can shop for health insurance coverage. These Marketplaces offer a range of qualified health plans with standardized coverage levels.

- **Essential Health Benefits:** The ACA mandates that health insurance plans must cover essential health benefits, including preventive services, maternity care, mental health services, prescription drugs, and more.

- **Pre-Existing Condition Coverage:** The ACA prohibits health insurance plans from denying coverage or charging higher premiums based on pre-existing conditions. This provision ensures individuals with pre-existing conditions can obtain and maintain health insurance coverage.

- **Dependent Coverage:** The ACA requires health insurance plans to allow young adults to stay on their parents' insurance plans until the age of 26, regardless of their student or employment status.

- **Medical Loss Ratio (MLR):** The ACA sets requirements for the MLR, which is the percentage of premium dollars that insurers must spend on medical care and healthcare quality improvement activities. Insurers must meet minimum MLR thresholds and provide rebates to policyholders if they fail to meet these thresholds.

- **Preventive Services:** The ACA mandates that health insurance plans cover certain preventive services, such as vaccinations, screenings, and counseling, without cost-sharing (e.g., co-payments, deductibles).

2. **Employee Retirement Income Security Act (ERISA):** ERISA is a federal law that sets standards for employee benefit plans, including health insurance plans provided by private employers. Key provisions of ERISA related to health insurance include:

   - **Plan Reporting and Disclosure:** ERISA requires employers to provide plan documents and summary plan descriptions to employees, outlining the terms, conditions, and coverage details of the health insurance plans.

   - **Fiduciary Duties:** ERISA imposes fiduciary responsibilities on plan administrators, requiring them to act in the best interests of plan participants and beneficiaries when managing the health insurance plan.

   - **Claims and Appeals Process:** ERISA establishes requirements for the claims and appeals process, ensuring that participants have the right to review and appeal denied claims and receive prompt and fair decisions.

   - **Nondiscrimination:** ERISA prohibits health insurance plans from discriminating against employees based on their health status, and it requires plans to offer continuation coverage (COBRA) to eligible individuals who lose their coverage due to specific events, such as termination of employment.

- **Preemption:** ERISA preempts certain state laws related to health insurance plans offered by employers, ensuring uniformity and consistency in the regulation of employee benefit plans.

Both the ACA and ERISA have had a significant impact on the health insurance landscape, shaping coverage options, consumer protections, and employer-sponsored health plans. Understanding these regulations is essential for insurance providers, employers, and individuals to navigate the health insurance market and ensure compliance with applicable laws. It's important to note that the specifics of these regulations can vary, and it's advisable to consult legal and regulatory resources for a comprehensive understanding of the requirements.

Compliance Requirements for Insurance Companies and Payers

Compliance requirements for insurance companies and payers are established to ensure ethical practices, consumer protection, and the fair and efficient operation of the insurance industry. These requirements vary based on jurisdiction and the type of insurance involved. Here are some common compliance requirements for insurance companies and payers:

1. **Licensing and Registration:** Insurance companies must obtain appropriate licenses or registrations from regulatory authorities to operate legally in a particular jurisdiction. The licensing process typically involves meeting specific criteria related to financial solvency, business integrity, and compliance with applicable laws and regulations.

2. **Financial Solvency and Reserves:** Insurance companies must maintain adequate financial reserves to fulfill their obligations to policyholders. Compliance requirements typically include periodic financial reporting, reserve calculations, and adherence to solvency ratios or other financial stability measures.

3. **Product Approval and Disclosure:** Insurance companies must comply with regulations related to product approval and disclosure. This includes submitting insurance policy forms for regulatory approval, providing

accurate and clear policy documentation to policyholders, and complying with guidelines for policy renewals, cancellations, and modifications.

4. **Rate Filing and Pricing:** Insurance companies are often required to file and justify premium rates with regulatory authorities. Compliance involves adhering to guidelines for rate setting, ensuring that rates are reasonable, non-discriminatory, and based on sound actuarial principles.

5. **Claims Handling and Settlement:** Insurance companies must have processes and procedures in place to handle claims promptly, fairly, and in accordance with applicable laws. Compliance requirements include accurate claims processing, timely claim settlement, claims investigation, and adherence to guidelines for claims disputes and appeals.

6. **Consumer Protection and Fair Practices:** Insurance companies must comply with consumer protection regulations and fair insurance practices. This includes provisions related to policyholder rights, privacy protection, marketing and sales practices, and disclosure of terms and conditions. Compliance efforts may involve implementing complaint resolution mechanisms and ensuring transparency in communication with policyholders.

7. **Network Adequacy and Provider Credentialing:** Payers are often required to maintain an adequate network of healthcare providers to ensure that policyholders have access to necessary healthcare services. Compliance involves evaluating and verifying provider credentials, monitoring network adequacy, and complying with regulations related to provider contracts, reimbursement rates, and timely access to care.

8. **Fraud and Abuse Prevention:** Insurance companies and payers must implement robust fraud detection and prevention programs to safeguard against fraudulent activities. Compliance requirements may include implementing fraud prevention measures, conducting audits and investigations, and participating in industry-wide fraud reporting initiatives.

9. **Data Privacy and Security:** Insurance companies must comply with data privacy and security regulations, such as the Health Insurance Portability and Accountability Act (HIPAA) and state-specific data protection laws. Compliance involves implementing safeguards to protect sensitive customer information, maintaining privacy policies, and responding appropriately to data breaches.

10. **Regulatory Reporting and Compliance Monitoring:** Insurance companies and payers are often required to submit regular reports and filings to regulatory authorities. Compliance efforts involve tracking and monitoring changes in regulations, staying up-to-date with compliance obligations, and maintaining accurate records and documentation.

Compliance requirements for insurance companies and payers may vary based on the type of insurance, such as health insurance, life insurance, or property and casualty insurance, and the jurisdiction in which they operate. It's important for insurance companies and payers to stay informed about applicable regulations, work closely with regulatory bodies, and establish robust compliance programs to ensure adherence to legal and ethical standards in their operations.

Ensuring Accurate Claims Processing and Reimbursement

Ensuring accurate claims processing and reimbursement is crucial for insurance companies and payers to maintain compliance, minimize errors, and provide timely and fair compensation to healthcare providers (Table 12.2). Here are some key strategies and considerations to ensure accurate claims processing and reimbursement:

▼ **Table 12.2:** Ensuring Accurate Claims Processing and Reimbursement

Compliance Measure	Description
Correct Coding and Billing	Ensuring accurate coding of medical procedures, services, and diagnoses, and proper billing practices.
Medical Documentation	Compliance with requirements for complete, accurate, and timely documentation to support claims and services.
Medical Necessity	Determining that services and procedures billed are reasonable and necessary for the patient's condition.
Claims Auditing and Monitoring	Regular auditing and monitoring of claims to identify billing errors, fraud, and compliance violations.

1. **Clear Claims Submission Guidelines:** Insurance companies and payers should establish clear and comprehensive guidelines for healthcare providers to submit claims. These guidelines should outline the required documentation,

coding standards (such as CPT and ICD codes), and any specific requirements for claim submission. Clear communication and education about these guidelines can help providers submit accurate and complete claims.

2. **Effective Claims Scrutiny and Validation:** Insurance companies and payers should employ robust claims scrutiny processes to validate the accuracy and completeness of submitted claims. This may include automated systems, manual reviews, or a combination of both. Claims should be checked for errors, such as missing information, incorrect coding, or inconsistent documentation. Advanced technologies, like artificial intelligence and machine learning, can be leveraged to enhance claims validation processes.

3. **Coding and Documentation Compliance:** Insurance companies and payers should ensure that healthcare providers adhere to coding and documentation compliance requirements. This includes using appropriate coding systems (such as CPT, ICD, and HCPCS) and documenting the medical necessity of services rendered. Regular provider education and feedback can help reinforce coding and documentation best practices.

4. **Transparent Reimbursement Policies:** Insurance companies and payers should establish transparent reimbursement policies that clearly define the reimbursement rates, billing methodologies, and any applicable fee schedules or payment schedules. Providers should have a clear understanding of how reimbursement amounts are calculated to avoid confusion or disputes.

5. **Timely Claims Adjudication:** Insurance companies and payers should strive for timely claims adjudication to ensure prompt payment to healthcare providers. Implementing efficient claims processing systems, utilizing electronic claims submission and adjudication platforms, and closely monitoring claims processing turnaround times can help expedite the reimbursement process.

6. **Provider Relations and Communication:** Establishing effective communication channels with healthcare providers is essential. Regular communication, such as provider newsletters, webinars, or dedicated provider relations representatives, can help clarify reimbursement policies, address provider concerns or questions, and promote collaboration in accurate claims processing.

7. **Claims Auditing and Internal Controls:** Insurance companies and payers should conduct periodic claims audits to assess the accuracy and compliance

of processed claims. Internal controls, such as random sampling, pre-payment and post-payment audits, and data analytics, can identify patterns of errors or potential fraudulent activities. Addressing identified issues promptly helps improve claims accuracy and prevent future discrepancies.

8. **Provider Education and Training:** Offering ongoing education and training programs to healthcare providers can enhance their understanding of claims submission requirements, coding guidelines, and documentation standards. This can include webinars, workshops, or online resources that focus on claims accuracy and compliance.

9. **Claims Dispute Resolution and Appeals:** Insurance companies and payers should establish clear processes for handling claims disputes and appeals. Providers should have access to a fair and transparent appeals process to address any disagreements regarding claim reimbursement. Timely and effective communication throughout the dispute resolution process is essential.

10. **Continuous Process Improvement:** Regularly reviewing claims processing workflows, analyzing data trends, and seeking feedback from healthcare providers can help identify areas for process improvement. Implementing technology solutions, streamlining administrative processes, and adopting best practices from industry benchmarks can optimize claims processing efficiency and accuracy.

By implementing these strategies and maintaining a strong focus on accuracy and compliance, insurance companies and payers can enhance the claims processing and reimbursement experience for healthcare providers, minimize errors, and foster positive relationships with their provider networks.

Ensuring Accurate Claims Processing and Reimbursement

Ensuring accurate claims processing and reimbursement is crucial for insurance companies and payers to maintain compliance, minimize errors, and provide timely and fair compensation to healthcare providers. Here are some key strategies and considerations to ensure accurate claims processing and reimbursement:

1. **Clear Claims Submission Guidelines:** Insurance companies and payers should establish clear and comprehensive guidelines for healthcare providers to submit claims. These guidelines should outline the required documentation,

coding standards (such as CPT and ICD codes), and any specific requirements for claim submission. Clear communication and education about these guidelines can help providers submit accurate and complete claims.

2. **Effective Claims Scrutiny and Validation:** Insurance companies and payers should employ robust claims scrutiny processes to validate the accuracy and completeness of submitted claims. This may include automated systems, manual reviews, or a combination of both. Claims should be checked for errors, such as missing information, incorrect coding, or inconsistent documentation. Advanced technologies, like artificial intelligence and machine learning, can be leveraged to enhance claims validation processes.

3. **Coding and Documentation Compliance:** Insurance companies and payers should ensure that healthcare providers adhere to coding and documentation compliance requirements. This includes using appropriate coding systems (such as CPT, ICD, and HCPCS) and documenting the medical necessity of services rendered. Regular provider education and feedback can help reinforce coding and documentation best practices.

4. **Transparent Reimbursement Policies:** Insurance companies and payers should establish transparent reimbursement policies that clearly define the reimbursement rates, billing methodologies, and any applicable fee schedules or payment schedules. Providers should have a clear understanding of how reimbursement amounts are calculated to avoid confusion or disputes.

5. **Timely Claims Adjudication:** Insurance companies and payers should strive for timely claims adjudication to ensure prompt payment to healthcare providers. Implementing efficient claims processing systems, utilizing electronic claims submission and adjudication platforms, and closely monitoring claims processing turnaround times can help expedite the reimbursement process.

6. **Provider Relations and Communication:** Establishing effective communication channels with healthcare providers is essential. Regular communication, such as provider newsletters, webinars, or dedicated provider relations representatives, can help clarify reimbursement policies, address provider concerns or questions, and promote collaboration in accurate claims processing.

7. **Claims Auditing and Internal Controls:** Insurance companies and payers should conduct periodic claims audits to assess the accuracy and compliance of processed claims. Internal controls, such as random

sampling, pre-payment and post-payment audits, and data analytics, can identify patterns of errors or potential fraudulent activities. Addressing identified issues promptly helps improve claims accuracy and prevent future discrepancies.

8. **Provider Education and Training:** Offering ongoing education and training programs to healthcare providers can enhance their understanding of claims submission requirements, coding guidelines, and documentation standards. This can include webinars, workshops, or online resources that focus on claims accuracy and compliance.

9. **Claims Dispute Resolution and Appeals:** Insurance companies and payers should establish clear processes for handling claims disputes and appeals. Providers should have access to a fair and transparent appeals process to address any disagreements regarding claim reimbursement. Timely and effective communication throughout the dispute resolution process is essential.

10. **Continuous Process Improvement:** Regularly reviewing claims processing workflows, analyzing data trends, and seeking feedback from healthcare providers can help identify areas for process improvement. Implementing technology solutions, streamlining administrative processes, and adopting best practices from industry benchmarks can optimize claims processing efficiency and accuracy.

By implementing these strategies and maintaining a strong focus on accuracy and compliance, insurance companies and payers can enhance the claims processing and reimbursement experience for healthcare providers, minimize errors, and foster positive relationships with their provider networks.

Addressing Compliance Challenges in Payer-provider Relationships

Payer-provider relationships in healthcare can be complex, with various compliance challenges that need to be addressed to ensure effective collaboration and adherence to regulatory requirements. Here are some strategies for addressing compliance challenges in payer-provider relationships:

1. **Transparent Contracting and Negotiations:** Establishing clear and transparent contractual agreements between payers and providers is crucial. Contracts should clearly outline reimbursement rates, payment

terms, service expectations, and compliance obligations. Open and collaborative negotiations can help ensure that both parties have a shared understanding of compliance requirements and can align their practices accordingly.

2. **Provider Network Adequacy:** Payers must ensure that their provider networks are adequate to meet the needs of their members. Compliance requires meeting regulatory requirements for network adequacy, such as geographic coverage, specialty availability, and appointment wait times. Regular assessments of network adequacy, provider credentialing, and ongoing monitoring can help address compliance challenges in maintaining a robust provider network.

3. **Claims Processing and Reimbursement:** Payers and providers must work together to ensure accurate claims processing and timely reimbursement. This involves clear communication of claims submission guidelines, coding and documentation requirements, and prompt resolution of claims disputes or inquiries. Collaboration in addressing claims-related compliance issues, such as coding errors or improper billing practices, helps foster accurate claims processing and proper reimbursement.

4. **Quality Reporting and Performance Metrics:** Compliance requirements often include quality reporting and performance metrics for providers. Payers should clearly communicate the quality metrics, reporting timelines, and data submission requirements to providers. Collaborating on data collection, validation, and reporting can help ensure accurate and timely compliance with quality reporting obligations.

5. **Data Sharing and Privacy:** Payers and providers must navigate data sharing and privacy regulations, such as HIPAA, when exchanging patient health information. Implementing appropriate data sharing agreements, ensuring secure data transmission, and maintaining patient privacy and confidentiality are crucial. Compliance efforts should focus on consent management, data access controls, and data breach prevention and response.

6. **Medical Necessity and Utilization Management:** Payers must implement utilization management programs to ensure the appropriate utilization of healthcare services and compliance with medical necessity requirements. Collaborating with providers to establish clear medical necessity guidelines, prior authorization processes, and communication channels can help address compliance challenges and foster mutual understanding.

7. **Provider Education and Communication:** Payers should provide ongoing education and support to providers on compliance requirements, changes in policies or procedures, and emerging industry trends. Regular communication channels, provider newsletters, webinars, and forums can facilitate knowledge sharing, clarify compliance expectations, and address provider concerns or questions.

8. **Auditing and Monitoring:** Payers and providers should conduct regular internal audits and monitoring activities to identify compliance gaps and mitigate potential risks. Auditing can include claims audits, documentation reviews, and assessments of compliance with contractual obligations. Collaboration in auditing and monitoring processes, sharing audit findings, and addressing areas of improvement helps strengthen compliance in payer-provider relationships.

9. **Dispute Resolution and Appeals:** Establishing fair and transparent processes for claims disputes, appeals, and grievances is essential. Payers and providers should communicate the steps, timelines, and documentation requirements for resolving disputes or appealing denied claims. Prompt and respectful communication throughout the resolution process can help address compliance challenges and maintain positive relationships.

10. **Collaboration in Regulatory Compliance:** Payers and providers should collaborate in addressing regulatory compliance requirements, such as those related to HIPAA, ACA, and fraud prevention. Sharing best practices, participating in compliance-related training, and engaging in industry initiatives and forums can enhance compliance knowledge and foster a culture of compliance in payer-provider relationships.

Addressing compliance challenges in payer-provider relationships requires open communication, collaboration, and a shared commitment to ethical practices and regulatory compliance. By working together, payers and providers can navigate the complexities of healthcare regulations, ensure quality care delivery, and build mutually beneficial relationships that prioritize patient outcomes and compliance with regulatory standards.

Chapter 13

Compliance in Long-term Care Facilities

Compliance in long-term care facilities is of paramount importance to ensure the safety, well-being, and quality of care for residents. Long-term care facilities, such as nursing homes, assisted living facilities, and skilled nursing facilities, must adhere to various regulatory requirements and industry standards. Here are key aspects of compliance in long-term care facilities:

1. **Licensing and Certification:** Long-term care facilities must obtain appropriate licenses and certifications from state regulatory agencies. Compliance requirements typically include meeting specific facility standards, staffing requirements, infection control protocols, and safety regulations. Regular inspections and surveys are conducted to ensure ongoing compliance.

2. **Resident Rights and Advocacy:** Compliance in long-term care facilities involves respecting and protecting the rights of residents. Facilities must comply with regulations that safeguard residents' rights to dignity, privacy, autonomy, and choice. This includes providing access to information, opportunities for participation in care planning, and processes for addressing grievances and resolving disputes.

3. **Quality of Care and Services:** Long-term care facilities must provide quality care and services that meet residents' physical, emotional, and social needs. Compliance efforts include implementing care plans, maintaining staffing levels, administering medications safely, preventing infections, managing pain, and addressing behavioral health needs. Compliance also involves ensuring staff competency through training and education.

4. **Safety and Environmental Compliance:** Long-term care facilities must maintain a safe and hazard-free environment for residents and staff. Compliance requirements include fire safety, emergency preparedness, infection control, proper handling of hazardous materials, and accessibility

for individuals with disabilities. Facilities must adhere to applicable federal, state, and local regulations and standards.

5. **Staffing and Training Compliance:** Adequate staffing levels and appropriate staff qualifications are critical for providing quality care in long-term care facilities. Compliance includes meeting state-mandated staffing ratios, ensuring staff are properly trained and licensed, conducting background checks, and implementing ongoing training and competency assessment programs for staff members.

6. **Resident Assessment and Care Planning:** Compliance involves conducting comprehensive assessments of residents upon admission and regularly reassessing their needs. Long-term care facilities must develop individualized care plans based on these assessments and regularly update them to reflect changes in residents' conditions. Compliance also includes involving residents and their families in the care planning process.

7. **Medication Management and Administration:** Long-term care facilities must have robust medication management systems in place to ensure accurate and safe administration of medications to residents. Compliance efforts include proper storage, documentation, and monitoring of medications, adherence to medication administration protocols, and implementation of medication reconciliation processes.

8. **Medical Records and Documentation:** Accurate and complete documentation is vital for compliance in long-term care facilities. Facilities must maintain comprehensive medical records that include residents' assessments, care plans, medication administration records, progress notes, and incident reports. Compliance requirements include adhering to documentation standards, confidentiality, and records retention policies.

9. **Infection Control and Prevention:** Long-term care facilities must have infection control programs to prevent and control the spread of infections. Compliance includes implementing standard precautions, educating staff on infection control practices, conducting surveillance for infections, and having policies and procedures in place for outbreak management and reporting.

10. **Ethics and Resident Rights Protection:** Long-term care facilities must adhere to ethical standards and protect residents from abuse, neglect, and exploitation. Compliance involves implementing policies and procedures for

resident rights protection, staff training on ethical conduct, and reporting and investigating allegations of abuse or neglect.

Compliance in long-term care facilities requires a comprehensive understanding of federal, state, and local regulations, as well as industry best practices. It involves ongoing monitoring, staff training and education, policy development, quality improvement initiatives, and collaboration with regulatory agencies to maintain a culture of compliance and ensure the well-being of residents.

Regulatory Considerations Specific to Long-term Care Facilities

Long-term care facilities are subject to specific regulatory considerations due to the unique nature of the care they provide. These regulations aim to ensure the safety, well-being, and quality of life for residents. Here are some regulatory considerations specific to long-term care facilities:

1. **Nursing Home Reform Act (OBRA '87):** The Nursing Home Reform Act, enacted under the Omnibus Budget Reconciliation Act of 1987 (OBRA '87), sets federal regulations for nursing homes participating in Medicare and Medicaid programs. It establishes standards for resident rights, quality of care, staffing, assessment, care planning, and facility services.

2. **Minimum Data Set (MDS) Assessments:** Long-term care facilities are required to conduct resident assessments using the Minimum Data Set (MDS) tool. The MDS assessment captures information about residents' physical, mental, and psychosocial well-being and forms the basis for care planning and quality measures reporting.

3. **Centers for Medicare and Medicaid Services (CMS) Regulations:** CMS, the federal agency that administers the Medicare and Medicaid programs, issues regulations and guidance specific to long-term care facilities. This includes the Conditions of Participation (COPs) for nursing homes, which outline the requirements for participation in these programs.

4. **State Licensing and Certification Regulations:** Long-term care facilities must comply with state-specific licensing and certification regulations. These regulations govern facility standards, staffing requirements, infection control protocols, safety measures, and other aspects of care. State regulatory agencies conduct inspections and surveys to assess compliance.

5. **Quality Assurance and Performance Improvement (QAPI):** Long-term care facilities are required to implement QAPI programs that focus on continuous quality improvement. QAPI programs involve data collection, analysis, and quality improvement activities to enhance resident care and safety.

6. **Resident Assessment Instrument (RAI) Process:** The RAI process, based on the MDS assessment, guides the comprehensive assessment of residents' functional abilities, medical conditions, and care needs. Compliance involves accurate and timely completion of the RAI process, including the MDS assessment, care area assessments, and the development of individualized care plans.

7. **Emergency Preparedness:** Long-term care facilities must have emergency preparedness plans in place to address potential disasters and emergencies. Compliance includes developing and implementing plans for evacuation, communication, sheltering-in-place, and coordination with local authorities.

8. **Staffing Ratios and Qualifications:** Long-term care facilities are subject to staffing requirements, including minimum staffing ratios and qualifications for licensed and non-licensed staff members. Compliance involves maintaining appropriate staffing levels and ensuring that staff meet the necessary qualifications and training requirements.

9. **Infection Control and Prevention:** Regulations specific to infection control and prevention are crucial in long-term care facilities. Compliance includes implementing infection control policies and procedures, conducting ongoing staff education and training, and adhering to guidelines for preventing healthcare-associated infections.

10. **Resident Rights and Advocacy:** Long-term care facilities must protect and uphold the rights of residents, including privacy, dignity, autonomy, and freedom from abuse and neglect. Compliance involves establishing policies and procedures to address resident rights, providing opportunities for resident participation and decision-making, and promptly addressing grievances and complaints.

These regulatory considerations are essential for long-term care facilities to ensure compliance, maintain quality care, and provide a safe and supportive environment for residents. Facilities must regularly review and update their policies, procedures, and practices to align with evolving regulations and best practices in long-term care.

Compliance with Nursing Home Regulations (CMS Guidelines, OIG Recommendations)

Compliance with nursing home regulations is crucial to ensure the safety, well-being, and quality of care for residents. Nursing homes must adhere to guidelines and recommendations provided by various regulatory bodies, including the Centers for Medicare and Medicaid Services (CMS) and the Office of Inspector General (OIG). Here's an overview of compliance considerations with nursing home regulations (Table 13.1):

▼ **Table 13.1:** Compliance with Nursing Home Regulations

Compliance Area	Description
Resident Rights	Ensuring residents' rights are respected and protected, including privacy, dignity, autonomy, and access to information and services.
Quality of Care	Providing high-quality care to residents, including medical, nursing, rehabilitation, and psychosocial services.
Staffing and Training	Maintaining appropriate staffing levels and ensuring staff members are properly trained to meet residents' needs.
Infection Control	Implementing infection control practices to prevent and control the spread of infectious diseases among residents and staff.

1. **Centers for Medicare and Medicaid Services (CMS) Guidelines:** CMS provides guidelines and regulations for nursing homes participating in Medicare and Medicaid programs. Some key areas of compliance include:

   - **Conditions of Participation (COPs):** Nursing homes must comply with the COPs outlined by CMS. These regulations cover various aspects of care, including resident rights, assessment and care planning, staffing requirements, infection control, quality assurance, and safety measures.

   - **Quality Reporting Programs:** Nursing homes are required to participate in quality reporting programs, such as the Nursing Home Quality Initiative (NHQI) and the Payroll-Based Journal (PBJ) system. Compliance involves accurate data reporting on measures such as resident assessments, staffing levels, quality indicators, and other performance metrics.

- **Survey and Certification Process:** Nursing homes undergo periodic surveys conducted by state survey agencies to assess compliance with CMS regulations. Compliance efforts involve preparing for surveys, addressing deficiencies identified during the survey process, and implementing corrective actions as necessary.

2. **Office of Inspector General (OIG) Recommendations:** The Office of Inspector General provides recommendations to improve program integrity, prevent fraud and abuse, and enhance the quality of care in nursing homes. Compliance considerations related to OIG recommendations include:

- **Fraud and Abuse Prevention:** Nursing homes should implement robust compliance programs to prevent and detect fraud, waste, and abuse. Compliance efforts include conducting internal audits, implementing fraud prevention measures, and educating staff on fraud awareness and reporting mechanisms.

- **Quality of Care and Resident Safety:** OIG recommendations often focus on improving the quality of care and resident safety in nursing homes. Compliance involves implementing best practices, following evidence-based guidelines, and addressing areas identified for improvement in OIG reports and recommendations.

- **Billing and Documentation:** OIG emphasizes accurate billing practices and proper documentation in nursing homes. Compliance includes ensuring proper coding, documentation of services provided, appropriate use of therapy services, and adherence to Medicare and Medicaid billing rules.

3. **Emergency Preparedness:** Nursing homes must comply with CMS regulations related to emergency preparedness. Compliance involves developing and implementing comprehensive emergency preparedness plans, conducting drills and exercises, and coordinating with local emergency response agencies.

4. **Staffing and Workforce Compliance:** Compliance with staffing regulations is essential to ensure adequate care for nursing home residents. Compliance efforts include meeting staffing requirements, ensuring appropriate staffing levels, and addressing staff training and competency needs.

5. **Infection Control and Prevention:** Nursing homes must have robust infection control programs to prevent and manage infections. Compliance includes implementing infection control protocols, providing staff education and training, conducting regular infection surveillance, and following guidelines from organizations such as the Centers for Disease Control and Prevention (CDC).

Compliance with nursing home regulations requires ongoing monitoring, staff education, policy development, and quality improvement initiatives. Nursing homes should stay updated with CMS guidelines and OIG recommendations, implement effective compliance programs, and collaborate with regulatory bodies to ensure the well-being of residents and maintain the highest standards of care.

Quality of Care and Resident Rights in Long-term Care Settings

Ensuring quality of care and protecting resident rights are paramount in long-term care settings. These aspects contribute to the overall well-being and dignity of residents. Here's an overview of quality of care and resident rights considerations in long-term care settings:

Quality of Care:

1. **Person-Centered Care:** Long-term care settings should prioritize person-centered care, tailoring services to meet the individual needs and preferences of residents. This involves involving residents in care planning, respecting their choices, and promoting their autonomy.

2. **Clinical Care and Treatment:** Long-term care facilities should provide appropriate clinical care and treatment to residents, including medical management, medication administration, wound care, pain management, and mental health support. Compliance involves adhering to evidence-based practices, professional standards, and regulations related to resident care.

3. **Staffing and Workforce:** Adequate staffing levels and appropriately trained staff are crucial for quality care. Compliance requires maintaining appropriate staffing ratios, ensuring staff have the necessary qualifications and training, and fostering a positive work environment that supports staff retention and job satisfaction.

4. **Fall Prevention and Safety:** Long-term care facilities should implement fall prevention programs to minimize the risk of resident falls. Compliance involves conducting fall risk assessments, implementing interventions, providing mobility aids, monitoring residents' safety, and maintaining a safe physical environment.

5. **Infection Control and Prevention:** Effective infection control practices are essential to protect residents from healthcare-associated infections. Compliance includes implementing infection control protocols, practicing hand hygiene, adhering to isolation precautions, monitoring infections, and promoting staff education and adherence to infection control guidelines.

6. **Nutrition and Hydration:** Long-term care facilities should ensure that residents receive adequate nutrition and hydration. Compliance involves offering nutritious meals and snacks, accommodating special dietary needs, monitoring residents' nutritional status, and promoting hydration to prevent dehydration.

Resident Rights:

1. **Dignity and Respect:** Long-term care settings must uphold residents' dignity and treat them with respect. Compliance involves training staff on respectful communication, promoting privacy during care activities, and addressing residents' preferences and cultural or religious beliefs.

2. **Informed Consent:** Residents have the right to make informed decisions about their care and treatment. Compliance requires obtaining informed consent for medical procedures, medication administration, participation in research, and other interventions. Facilities should ensure residents understand the risks, benefits, and alternatives before consenting.

3. **Privacy and Confidentiality:** Residents' privacy and confidentiality must be protected. Compliance includes maintaining the confidentiality of health information, providing private spaces for conversations and examinations, and implementing safeguards for resident privacy, such as ensuring that personal information is not shared without consent.

4. **Freedom from Abuse and Neglect:** Residents have the right to live free from abuse, neglect, and exploitation. Compliance involves implementing policies and procedures to prevent and address abuse, promptly reporting incidents,

conducting investigations, and providing staff training on recognizing and reporting abuse.

5. **Grievance Procedures:** Long-term care facilities should have established grievance procedures for residents to voice concerns or complaints. Compliance requires providing residents with information about the grievance process, investigating grievances promptly, and taking appropriate action to address valid complaints.

6. **Visitation Rights:** Residents have the right to receive visitors and maintain relationships with family and friends. Compliance involves allowing reasonable visitation hours, accommodating visitors, and respecting residents' preferences regarding visitation.

Ensuring quality of care and protecting resident rights requires a commitment from long-term care facilities to implement policies, train staff, promote person-centered care, and regularly assess and improve the care provided. Compliance with regulations and adherence to best practices are crucial to fostering a supportive and respectful environment for residents in long-term care settings.

Challenges and Best Practices for Maintaining Compliance in Long-term Care Facilities

Maintaining compliance in long-term care facilities can be challenging due to the complex regulatory environment and the unique needs of the resident population. However, adopting best practices can help overcome these challenges and promote a culture of compliance. Here are some common challenges and best practices for maintaining compliance in long-term care facilities:

Challenges:

1. **Complex Regulatory Landscape:** Long-term care facilities must navigate numerous federal, state, and local regulations, which can be complex and subject to frequent changes. Staying updated with regulatory requirements and interpreting them correctly is a significant challenge.

2. **Staffing Shortages and Turnover:** Adequate staffing is crucial for providing quality care and maintaining compliance. Staffing shortages and high turnover rates can strain the ability to ensure consistent adherence to regulations and quality standards.

3. **Training and Education:** Comprehensive training and ongoing education for staff are essential for maintaining compliance. However, allocating resources for training programs and keeping staff updated on evolving regulations can be challenging.

4. **Data Management and Reporting:** Compliance often involves accurate data management, reporting, and documentation. Facilities may face challenges in ensuring consistent and accurate data collection, maintaining electronic health records, and meeting reporting deadlines.

5. **Budget Constraints:** Limited financial resources can pose challenges in implementing and maintaining compliance programs, conducting necessary audits, and investing in staff training and technology upgrades.

Best Practices:

1. **Robust Compliance Program:** Establish a comprehensive compliance program that includes policies, procedures, and processes to ensure adherence to regulations. This includes designating a compliance officer, conducting regular compliance audits, and providing staff training on compliance requirements.

2. **Stay Informed and Updated:** Stay abreast of regulatory changes and industry best practices by actively monitoring updates from regulatory agencies, participating in industry associations, attending conferences, and leveraging resources from reputable sources.

3. **Staff Education and Training:** Invest in ongoing education and training programs for staff to enhance their understanding of regulations, compliance obligations, and best practices. Provide training on resident rights, infection control, documentation requirements, and ethical conduct.

4. **Effective Communication and Collaboration:** Foster open communication and collaboration among staff, residents, families, and regulatory agencies. Establish mechanisms for reporting compliance concerns, addressing grievances, and implementing feedback loops to identify areas for improvement.

5. **Quality Assurance and Performance Improvement (QAPI):** Implement a robust QAPI program that focuses on continuous quality improvement and compliance. Monitor key performance indicators, conduct regular internal audits, identify areas for improvement, and develop action plans to address deficiencies.

6. **Engage Residents and Families:** Involve residents and their families in care planning, decision-making, and quality improvement initiatives. Encourage feedback, conduct resident satisfaction surveys, and address concerns promptly to enhance resident-centered care and compliance.

7. **Effective Documentation and Record-Keeping:** Emphasize accurate and complete documentation practices, including comprehensive resident assessments, care plans, and incident reports. Implement electronic health records systems to improve documentation accuracy, accessibility, and data management.

8. **Audit and Monitoring Programs:** Develop robust audit and monitoring programs to identify compliance gaps, detect potential issues, and implement corrective actions. Regularly assess adherence to policies, procedures, and regulatory requirements through internal audits and external assessments.

9. **Continuous Staff Engagement:** Foster a culture of compliance by engaging staff in the compliance process. Encourage staff to report potential compliance concerns, provide opportunities for staff input on compliance initiatives, and recognize and reward staff contributions to maintaining compliance.

10. **Collaboration with Regulatory Agencies:** Establish open lines of communication and collaborate with regulatory agencies. Proactively engage with surveyors during inspections, respond promptly to deficiencies, and maintain a cooperative relationship to address compliance issues effectively.

By implementing these best practices, long-term care facilities can navigate compliance challenges more effectively, ensure resident safety and well-being, and uphold the highest standards of care. These practices promote a culture of compliance, support ongoing quality improvement, and foster positive relationships with residents, staff, families, and regulatory agencies.

Compliance and Healthcare Fraud Investigations

Compliance plays a crucial role in preventing and detecting healthcare fraud, waste, and abuse. Healthcare fraud investigations are conducted to identify fraudulent activities, recover funds, and hold individuals or entities accountable for fraudulent practices. Here's an overview of the relationship between compliance and healthcare fraud investigations:

Compliance and Fraud Prevention:

1. **Effective Compliance Programs:** Robust compliance programs are essential in preventing healthcare fraud. These programs include policies, procedures, and internal controls that promote adherence to laws, regulations, and ethical standards. By implementing comprehensive compliance measures, organizations can proactively identify and address potential fraudulent activities.

2. **Education and Training:** Compliance programs should include training and education for staff on recognizing and preventing fraud, waste, and abuse. Training sessions can focus on identifying fraudulent schemes, understanding applicable laws and regulations, and reporting suspicious activities. Educating employees about compliance expectations fosters a culture of integrity and ethical behavior.

3. **Monitoring and Auditing:** Regular monitoring and auditing of healthcare operations help identify compliance weaknesses and potential fraud indicators. These processes involve reviewing claims, coding practices, billing patterns, and other data to detect irregularities or suspicious activities. Monitoring can be conducted internally or through external audits by specialized organizations.

4. **Internal Reporting Mechanisms:** Compliance programs should establish confidential reporting mechanisms, such as hotlines or reporting portals,

to encourage employees, contractors, and others to report suspected fraudulent activities. Whistleblower protection policies can also be implemented to safeguard individuals who report in good faith.

Healthcare Fraud Investigations:

1. **Investigative Authorities:** Various government agencies are responsible for investigating healthcare fraud, such as the Office of Inspector General (OIG), the Department of Justice (DOJ), and state Medicaid Fraud Control Units (MFCUs). These agencies have the authority to conduct civil, administrative, or criminal investigations, and they collaborate with law enforcement agencies to uncover fraudulent activities.

2. **Data Analysis and Intelligence:** Healthcare fraud investigations often involve data analysis and the use of sophisticated technologies to identify patterns, anomalies, and trends that may indicate fraudulent activities. Advanced data analytics can help identify unusual billing patterns, inappropriate coding practices, or suspicious provider behavior.

3. **Collaboration and Information Sharing:** Investigators collaborate with various stakeholders, including government agencies, law enforcement entities, regulatory bodies, and industry partners, to share information and gather evidence during investigations. Effective communication and collaboration facilitate the exchange of information needed to detect and investigate healthcare fraud.

4. **Audits and Reviews:** Investigators conduct audits and reviews of healthcare providers, suppliers, and entities suspected of fraudulent activities. These audits can involve reviewing medical records, financial documents, claims data, and billing practices to identify fraudulent billing, up-coding, kickbacks, or other fraudulent schemes.

5. **Prosecution and Enforcement:** Upon completing a healthcare fraud investigation, law enforcement agencies may initiate legal action against individuals or entities involved in fraudulent activities. This can lead to civil or criminal charges, fines, restitution, and exclusion from government healthcare programs.

Compliance and Collaboration with Investigations:

1. **Compliance Reporting:** Compliance programs should have mechanisms in place for reporting suspected fraud or misconduct internally. Prompt

reporting of potential fraud allows organizations to investigate the matter and cooperate with law enforcement agencies as necessary.

2. **Responding to Investigations:** In the event of a healthcare fraud investigation, organizations must cooperate fully with the investigative authorities. This includes providing requested documentation, facilitating interviews, and addressing any identified compliance deficiencies or fraudulent activities.

3. **Remediation and Corrective Actions:** If fraudulent activities are identified during an investigation, organizations should take immediate action to address the issue, implement corrective measures, and strengthen their compliance programs to prevent future occurrences. Cooperation and remediation efforts can demonstrate a commitment to compliance and mitigation of fraudulent activities.

4. **Ongoing Compliance Enhancement:**

   Healthcare fraud investigations serve as opportunities for organizations to learn from identified vulnerabilities and strengthen their compliance efforts. Organizations should use the findings from investigations to enhance their compliance programs, improve internal controls, and implement additional training and monitoring measures to prevent similar fraud schemes in the future.

Compliance and healthcare fraud investigations are interconnected in the effort to safeguard the healthcare system from fraudulent activities. Effective compliance programs help prevent and detect healthcare fraud, while investigations aim to identify and hold accountable those involved in fraudulent practices. By promoting a culture of compliance, organizations can actively contribute to the prevention of healthcare fraud and support the integrity of the healthcare industry.

Overview of Healthcare Fraud and Abuse Investigations

Healthcare fraud and abuse investigations are conducted to identify and address fraudulent activities, waste, and abuse within the healthcare system. These investigations aim to protect public funds, ensure the integrity of healthcare programs, and hold individuals and entities accountable for their actions. Here's an overview of healthcare fraud and abuse investigations (Figure 14.1):

Types of Healthcare Fraud and Abuse:

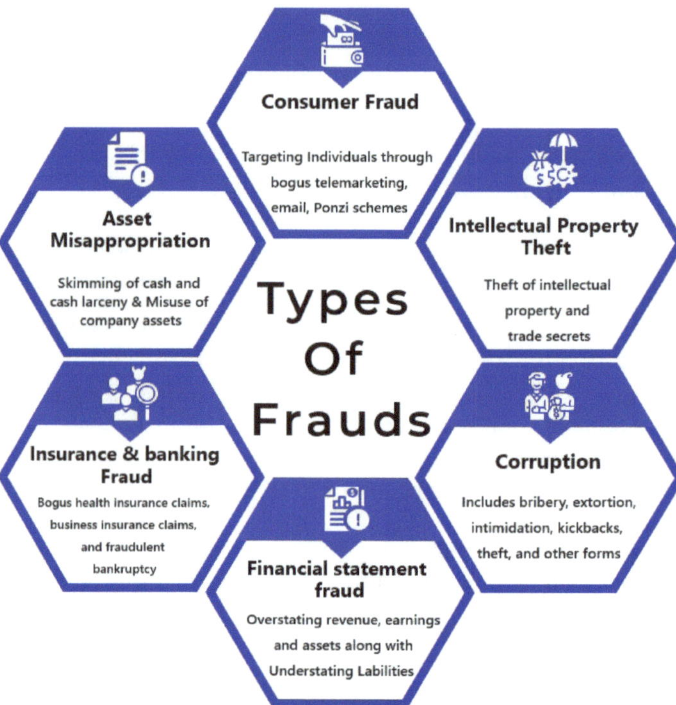

▼ **Figure 14.1:** Types of Fraud

1. **Billing Fraud:** Billing fraud involves intentionally submitting false or misleading claims for healthcare services or supplies. This can include up-coding (billing for a higher level of service than provided), unbundling (billing separately for services that should be billed together), and billing for services not provided.

2. **Kickbacks and Illegal Referrals:** Kickbacks occur when healthcare providers receive payment or other benefits in exchange for patient referrals or the purchase of goods or services. Illegal referrals involve referring patients to facilities or providers with whom there is a financial relationship, violating anti-kickback laws.

3. **Pharmaceutical Fraud:** Pharmaceutical fraud includes activities such as off-label marketing (promoting a drug for uses not approved by regulatory authorities), fraudulent claims for prescription drugs, and illegal promotion of prescription medications.

4. **Identity Theft:** Identity theft occurs when individuals' personal information, such as Medicare or Medicaid numbers, is unlawfully obtained and used to submit fraudulent claims or obtain services or supplies.

5. **Home Healthcare Fraud:** Home healthcare fraud involves billing for unnecessary services, falsifying patient records, and providing substandard care to patients receiving home healthcare services.

6. **Medical Equipment Fraud:** This type of fraud includes fraudulent billing for durable medical equipment, prosthetics, orthotics, and supplies that were not necessary or not provided to patients.

Investigative Agencies and Processes:

1. **Office of Inspector General (OIG):** The OIG is responsible for investigating fraud and abuse within the U.S. Department of Health and Human Services (HHS) programs, including Medicare and Medicaid. The OIG conducts investigations, audits, and evaluations to identify and address fraudulent activities.

2. **Department of Justice (DOJ):** The DOJ has jurisdiction to investigate and prosecute healthcare fraud cases involving federal programs, such as Medicare and Medicaid. It works closely with the OIG and other law enforcement agencies to investigate and bring legal action against perpetrators of healthcare fraud.

3. **Medicaid Fraud Control Units (MFCUs):** MFCUs are state-level agencies dedicated to investigating and prosecuting Medicaid fraud and abuse. They collaborate with federal agencies and state law enforcement to uncover fraudulent activities, recover funds, and hold individuals accountable.

4. **Data Analysis and Review:** Investigators use advanced data analysis techniques and tools to identify patterns, anomalies, and outliers that may indicate fraudulent activities. This involves analyzing billing data, claims data, medical records, and other relevant information to identify potential fraud schemes.

5. **Whistleblower Complaints:** Investigations may be initiated based on whistleblower complaints filed by individuals with knowledge of fraudulent activities. Whistleblowers, protected by the False Claims Act, can provide valuable information and evidence to support investigations.

6. **Cooperation with Law Enforcement:** Investigative agencies collaborate with law enforcement entities, including the Federal Bureau of Investigation (FBI) and state and local law enforcement agencies, to gather evidence, conduct interviews, and build cases against individuals or entities suspected of healthcare fraud.

Outcomes and Penalties:

Healthcare fraud and abuse investigations can result in various outcomes and penalties, depending on the severity and extent of the fraudulent activities:

1. **Civil and Criminal Prosecutions:** Investigations may lead to civil or criminal charges against individuals or entities involved in healthcare fraud. Penalties can include fines, imprisonment, restitution, and exclusion from government healthcare programs.

2. **Settlements and Repayment:** Perpetrators of healthcare fraud may enter into settlement agreements with investigative agencies, agreeing to repay funds obtained through fraudulent activities. These settlements often include additional penalties and obligations, such as implementing compliance programs or undergoing independent monitoring.

3. **Exclusion from Healthcare Programs:** Individuals or entities found guilty of healthcare fraud may be excluded from participating in Medicare, Medicaid, and other government healthcare programs. Exclusion prohibits them from billing or providing services reimbursed by these programs.

4. **Recovery of Funds:** Investigative agencies work to recover funds lost to fraudulent activities. This can involve seizing assets, freezing bank accounts, and pursuing restitution to reimburse government healthcare programs for fraudulent claims.

5. **Corporate Integrity Agreements (CIAs):** In cases involving corporate entities, CIAs may be imposed as part of a settlement or resolution. CIAs outline specific obligations, including enhanced compliance measures, independent monitoring, and reporting requirements to prevent future fraudulent activities.

Healthcare fraud and abuse investigations are crucial to protect public funds, maintain the integrity of healthcare programs, and ensure quality care for patients. By identifying and addressing fraudulent activities, these investigations help maintain trust in the healthcare system and promote the efficient and appropriate use of healthcare resources.

Role of Government Agencies (DOJ, OIG) in Enforcing Compliance

Government agencies, such as the Department of Justice (DOJ) and the Office of Inspector General (OIG), play a vital role in enforcing compliance within the healthcare industry. These agencies are responsible for investigating and prosecuting healthcare fraud, waste, and abuse, as well as ensuring compliance with applicable laws and regulations. Here's an overview of the roles of the DOJ and the OIG in enforcing compliance:

Department of Justice (DOJ):

1. **Civil and Criminal Investigations:** The DOJ conducts civil and criminal investigations into healthcare fraud and abuse cases. This includes investigating individuals, organizations, and entities suspected of fraudulent activities, such as submitting false claims, engaging in kickbacks, or participating in other fraudulent schemes.

2. **Prosecution:** The DOJ has the authority to prosecute individuals and entities involved in healthcare fraud. Through its Criminal Division and United States Attorneys' Offices, the DOJ brings criminal charges against perpetrators, seeking convictions and appropriate penalties, including fines and imprisonment.

3. **False Claims Act (FCA) Enforcement:** The DOJ plays a significant role in enforcing the False Claims Act, which prohibits knowingly submitting false or fraudulent claims to the government. The DOJ can initiate FCA lawsuits, intervene in whistleblower cases, and negotiate settlements or judgments to recover funds obtained through fraudulent activities.

4. **Coordination with Law Enforcement:** The DOJ collaborates with other law enforcement agencies, including the Federal Bureau of Investigation (FBI), to investigate healthcare fraud cases. This coordination allows for the pooling of resources, expertise, and information to build strong cases against perpetrators of healthcare fraud.

Office of Inspector General (OIG):

1. **Investigations and Audits:** The OIG conducts investigations, audits, and evaluations to uncover fraud, waste, and abuse within the Department of Health and Human Services (HHS) programs, including Medicare and

Medicaid. The OIG has broad investigative authority and can initiate cases based on referrals, data analysis, whistleblower complaints, and its own findings.

2. **Civil and Administrative Actions:** The OIG can pursue civil and administrative actions against individuals and entities involved in healthcare fraud and abuse. This includes imposing civil monetary penalties, excluding individuals or entities from participating in federal healthcare programs, and negotiating settlements to resolve allegations.

3. **Guidance and Compliance Oversight:** The OIG provides guidance and publishes compliance program guidance for healthcare organizations to help prevent fraud and abuse. The OIG also conducts compliance program reviews and assessments to evaluate the effectiveness of compliance efforts within healthcare entities.

4. **Provider Self-Disclosure Programs:** The OIG offers self-disclosure programs that allow healthcare providers to voluntarily report and resolve potential violations of laws and regulations. These programs provide incentives for self-disclosure, cooperation, and repayment, potentially reducing the severity of penalties.

5. **Advisory Opinions:** The OIG issues advisory opinions that provide guidance on the interpretation and application of healthcare fraud and abuse laws. These opinions help healthcare providers and entities understand the OIG's perspective on specific compliance matters and potential risks.

Both the DOJ and the OIG collaborate closely with other government agencies, including state Medicaid Fraud Control Units (MFCUs) and regulatory bodies, to enhance enforcement efforts and promote compliance in the healthcare industry. Their actions serve to protect public funds, deter fraudulent activities, and ensure the integrity and sustainability of government healthcare programs.

Whistleblower Protections and the False Claims Act

Whistleblower protections and the False Claims Act (FCA) are critical components in combating healthcare fraud and encouraging individuals to come forward with information about fraudulent activities. These protections provide legal safeguards and incentives for whistleblowers to report fraud and assist in enforcing compliance. Here's an overview of whistleblower protections and the role of the False Claims Act:

Whistleblower Protections:

1. **False Claims Act (FCA) Qui Tam Provisions:** The FCA includes qui tam provisions that allow individuals, known as whistleblowers or relators, to file lawsuits on behalf of the government against individuals or entities engaged in fraudulent activities. Whistleblowers who file qui tam lawsuits are entitled to a percentage of any recovered funds as a reward.

2. **Anti-Retaliation Provisions:** Whistleblower protection laws, such as the Whistleblower Protection Act and the Sarbanes-Oxley Act, prohibit retaliation against individuals who report fraudulent activities. Retaliation can include termination, demotion, harassment, or other adverse actions. Whistleblowers who experience retaliation may be entitled to remedies, including reinstatement, back pay, and compensation for damages.

3. **Confidentiality and Anonymity:** Whistleblower protection laws allow individuals to report fraud confidentially or anonymously to protect their identity. This ensures that individuals who fear retaliation can provide valuable information without exposing themselves to personal or professional risks.

4. **Whistleblower Reward Programs:** Government agencies, such as the Department of Justice (DOJ) and the Securities and Exchange Commission (SEC), have established reward programs to incentivize whistleblowers to come forward. Whistleblowers who provide original information leading to successful enforcement actions can receive a percentage of the recovered funds as a reward.

The False Claims Act (FCA):

1. **FCA Liability for False Claims:** The False Claims Act imposes liability on individuals or entities that knowingly submit false or fraudulent claims for payment to the government. This includes submitting false claims to Medicare, Medicaid, and other federal healthcare programs. Violators can be held accountable for damages, civil penalties, and treble damages (up to three times the government's actual damages).

2. **Qui Tam Lawsuits:** The FCA allows private individuals, or whistleblowers, to file qui tam lawsuits on behalf of the government. Whistleblowers can bring lawsuits against individuals or entities believed to have defrauded the government by submitting false claims. If the lawsuit is successful, the whistleblower may receive a portion (typically 15-30%) of the recovered funds as a reward.

3. **Government Intervention and Enforcement:** After a qui tam lawsuit is filed, the government has the option to intervene and take over the case. If the government decides not to intervene, the whistleblower may pursue the lawsuit independently. Even if the government does not intervene, the whistleblower can still receive a reward if the lawsuit is successful.

4. **Investigations and Penalties:** The FCA empowers government agencies, such as the Department of Justice (DOJ), to investigate alleged violations. The DOJ can initiate civil or criminal investigations, gather evidence, and negotiate settlements or pursue litigation to recover funds and hold violators accountable. Penalties under the FCA can include fines, treble damages, and exclusion from government healthcare programs.

The FCA and whistleblower protections serve as powerful tools in detecting and deterring healthcare fraud. They encourage individuals with knowledge of fraudulent activities to come forward, provide valuable information, and assist in enforcing compliance. These protections help safeguard public funds, maintain the integrity of healthcare programs, and hold accountable those engaged in fraudulent practices.

Responding to Investigations and Managing Legal Implications

When facing an investigation, healthcare organizations must respond effectively to protect their interests, manage legal implications, and cooperate with the investigating authorities. Here are some key considerations for responding to investigations and managing legal implications:

1. **Internal Assessment:** Conduct an internal assessment to gather relevant information and assess the scope and nature of the investigation. Identify the individuals involved, gather relevant documents and records, and determine potential areas of concern or violations.

2. **Legal Counsel:** Engage experienced legal counsel specializing in healthcare compliance and investigations. Legal counsel can provide guidance on the organization's rights and obligations, assist in formulating a response strategy, and communicate with the investigating authorities on behalf of the organization.

3. **Preservation of Documents:** Implement a legal hold on all relevant documents, records, and data to ensure their preservation. This includes

electronic records, emails, financial records, contracts, and any other documentation related to the investigation.

4. **Cooperation with Investigating Authorities:** Cooperate fully with the investigating authorities while working closely with legal counsel. Respond promptly to information requests, subpoenas, or interviews, and provide accurate and complete information as required. However, it is important to consult legal counsel before providing any information or engaging in discussions with investigators.

5. **Legal Privilege:** Understand and assert any applicable legal privileges, such as attorney-client privilege or work product doctrine, to protect confidential communications and legal strategies. Consult legal counsel to determine the applicability of these privileges and to guide the organization on preserving and asserting them.

6. **Internal Investigation:** Consider conducting an internal investigation to uncover any potential compliance deficiencies or violations. This internal investigation should be conducted under the guidance of legal counsel to maintain privilege, ensure independence, and identify areas of concern that need remediation.

7. **Remediation and Corrective Actions:** If compliance deficiencies or violations are identified, take prompt and appropriate remedial actions. This may include implementing corrective measures, revising policies and procedures, providing additional training, or strengthening internal controls to prevent future violations.

8. **Communication and Public Relations:** Develop a communication strategy to address inquiries from employees, patients, stakeholders, and the media. Ensure that all communications are consistent, transparent, and compliant with legal requirements. Consult with legal counsel and public relations experts to effectively manage the organization's reputation during the investigation.

9. **Legal Resolution:** If the investigation leads to legal proceedings or settlement discussions, work closely with legal counsel to evaluate the organization's options and develop a strategy for resolution. This may involve negotiating settlements, entering into corporate integrity agreements, or contesting allegations through litigation, depending on the circumstances.

10. **Monitor Compliance Program:** After the investigation, review and strengthen the organization's compliance program to address any identified

weaknesses and prevent future compliance issues. Regularly assess and monitor the effectiveness of the compliance program to ensure ongoing compliance with applicable laws and regulations.

Navigating investigations and managing legal implications require a coordinated approach with legal counsel, internal stakeholders, and compliance professionals. By responding appropriately, cooperating with investigating authorities, and taking remedial actions, healthcare organizations can mitigate legal risks, protect their interests, and demonstrate a commitment to compliance and integrity.

Compliance Auditing and Monitoring

ompliance auditing and monitoring are essential components of an effective compliance program in healthcare organizations. These processes help assess adherence to applicable laws, regulations, and internal policies, identify areas of non-compliance, and implement corrective actions. Here's an overview of compliance auditing and monitoring (Figure 15.1):

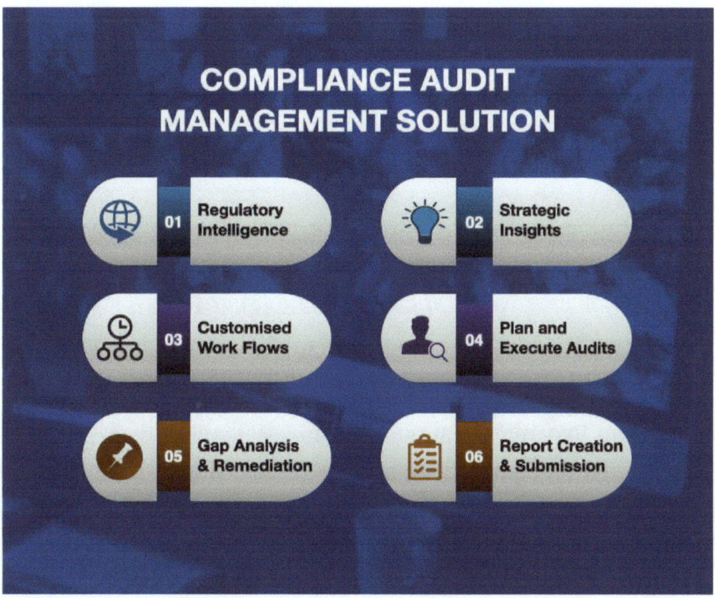

▼ **Figure 15.1:** Compliance Auditing

Compliance Auditing:

1. **Objective Assessment:** Compliance auditing involves the systematic and objective assessment of an organization's operations, processes, and practices to determine compliance with applicable laws and regulations. It aims to identify gaps, risks, and areas of non-compliance.

2. **Internal or External Audits:** Audits can be conducted internally by a dedicated compliance team or externally by independent auditors or consultants. External audits may bring fresh perspectives and specialized expertise, while internal audits allow for ongoing monitoring and familiarity with the organization's operations.

3. **Risk-Based Approach:** Compliance audits should be conducted using a risk-based approach, focusing on areas with a higher risk of non-compliance or where regulatory changes have occurred. Risk assessments help prioritize audit activities and allocate resources effectively.

4. **Compliance Program Evaluation:** Audits assess the effectiveness of the compliance program itself, including the design, implementation, and ongoing management of policies, procedures, training, and monitoring activities. This evaluation helps identify areas for improvement in the compliance program.

5. **Sampling and Testing:** Auditors select a representative sample of transactions, documents, or processes for detailed review and testing. This provides an understanding of the organization's compliance practices, identifies errors or inconsistencies, and determines the overall level of compliance.

6. **Documentation Review:** Auditors review relevant documents, such as policies, procedures, contracts, billing records, and employee files, to assess compliance with applicable regulations and internal guidelines. Documentation review helps identify gaps in record-keeping, improper documentation practices, or incomplete information.

7. **Findings and Recommendations:** Auditors document their findings, including instances of non-compliance, potential risks, and areas for improvement. They provide recommendations for corrective actions and enhancements to strengthen compliance practices.

Compliance Monitoring:

1. **Ongoing Oversight:** Compliance monitoring is a continuous process that involves ongoing oversight of key compliance areas. It focuses on tracking and reviewing compliance indicators, monitoring internal controls, and identifying emerging compliance risks.

2. **Key Performance Indicators (KPIs):** Monitoring involves establishing KPIs or metrics to measure and track compliance performance. These indicators can

include claims denial rates, billing error rates, employee training completion rates, whistleblower hotline reports, and other relevant metrics.

3. **Data Analytics:** Monitoring activities often leverage data analytics tools and technologies to identify patterns, trends, and anomalies that may indicate compliance issues. Advanced data analytics help analyze large volumes of data and detect potential fraud, waste, or abuse.

4. **Compliance Reporting:** Monitoring involves regular reporting on compliance activities and findings to management and the compliance officer. Reporting may include summaries of monitoring activities, key findings, remediation efforts, and trends in compliance performance.

5. **Corrective Actions and Follow-up:** Monitoring activities identify areas of non-compliance or weaknesses in internal controls. Organizations should promptly initiate corrective actions to address identified issues, and monitoring should track the implementation and effectiveness of these actions.

6. **Continuous Improvement:** Compliance monitoring supports a culture of continuous improvement by identifying areas for enhancement, evaluating the effectiveness of compliance initiatives, and adjusting compliance strategies based on evolving risks and regulatory changes.

By conducting regular compliance audits and implementing ongoing monitoring processes, healthcare organizations can proactively identify compliance gaps, address non-compliance, and continuously improve their compliance programs. These activities help mitigate risks, ensure adherence to applicable regulations, and promote a culture of integrity and compliance throughout the organization.

Importance of Regular Auditing and Monitoring in Compliance Programs

Regular auditing and monitoring play a crucial role in the effectiveness of compliance programs in healthcare organizations. Here are some reasons highlighting the importance of regular auditing and monitoring:

1. **Identifying Non-Compliance:** Auditing and monitoring activities help identify areas of non-compliance with laws, regulations, and internal policies. By systematically reviewing operations, processes, and practices, organizations can detect deviations, errors, or gaps in compliance and take corrective actions promptly.

2. **Risk Identification and Mitigation:** Regular auditing and monitoring allow organizations to assess and mitigate compliance risks. By proactively identifying areas with a higher risk of non-compliance, organizations can focus their resources on implementing preventive measures, strengthening internal controls, and reducing the likelihood of compliance breaches.

3. **Enhancing Operational Efficiency:** Auditing and monitoring processes also contribute to operational efficiency by identifying process inefficiencies, bottlenecks, or duplication of efforts. Through audits, organizations can identify opportunities for streamlining processes, improving documentation, and implementing best practices that align with compliance requirements.

4. **Preventing Fraud and Abuse:** Auditing and monitoring activities are instrumental in detecting and preventing fraud, waste, and abuse. By analyzing financial records, claims data, and billing practices, organizations can identify fraudulent patterns, improper billing, or fraudulent schemes, protecting both financial resources and the integrity of healthcare programs.

5. **Assessing Compliance Program Effectiveness:** Regular auditing and monitoring provide insights into the effectiveness of the compliance program itself. By evaluating the design, implementation, and ongoing management of compliance policies, training programs, and internal controls, organizations can identify areas for improvement and make necessary adjustments to ensure the compliance program's effectiveness.

6. **Demonstrating Regulatory Compliance:** Auditing and monitoring activities generate documentation and evidence of the organization's commitment to compliance. This documentation can be used to demonstrate compliance with regulatory requirements, respond to inquiries from regulatory bodies, and fulfill reporting obligations.

7. **Detecting Emerging Compliance Risks:** Healthcare regulations are constantly evolving, and new compliance risks may emerge. Regular auditing and monitoring help organizations stay vigilant and adapt to emerging compliance risks. By monitoring industry trends, regulatory updates, and internal data, organizations can proactively address emerging risks and update their compliance programs accordingly.

8. **Promoting a Culture of Compliance:** Regular auditing and monitoring foster a culture of compliance within the organization. Employees become aware that compliance is a priority, and accountability for adherence to policies and regulations is emphasized. This culture promotes ethical behavior, integrity, and responsibility throughout the organization.

In summary, regular auditing and monitoring are essential components of effective compliance programs in healthcare organizations. They provide organizations with a proactive approach to identify non-compliance, mitigate risks, enhance operational efficiency, prevent fraud and abuse, assess program effectiveness, and promote a culture of compliance. By incorporating these activities into their compliance efforts, organizations can ensure regulatory compliance, protect their reputation, and maintain the highest standards of integrity in delivering healthcare services.

Developing an Effective Auditing and Monitoring Framework

Developing an effective auditing and monitoring framework is crucial for healthcare organizations to ensure regulatory compliance and mitigate risks. Here are key steps to consider when developing such a framework:

1. **Assess Regulatory Requirements:** Begin by understanding the applicable regulatory requirements, industry standards, and best practices related to auditing and monitoring in healthcare. Identify the specific regulations and guidelines that impact your organization, such as those from government agencies like the Office of Inspector General (OIG) and Centers for Medicare and Medicaid Services (CMS).

2. **Define Objectives and Scope:** Clearly define the objectives of your auditing and monitoring framework. Determine the scope of the framework, including the areas, processes, and functions to be audited and monitored. Consider critical areas such as billing and coding, documentation practices, patient safety, privacy and security, and contractual compliance.

3. **Risk Assessment:** Conduct a comprehensive risk assessment to identify compliance risks and prioritize areas for auditing and monitoring. Evaluate both internal and external factors that may impact compliance, such as regulatory changes, organizational structure, vendor relationships, and previous audit findings. Focus on high-risk areas where non-compliance poses significant financial, legal, or reputational risks.

4. **Establish Compliance Policies and Procedures:** Develop clear policies and procedures that outline the auditing and monitoring activities, methodologies, and protocols to be followed. Ensure that the policies align with regulatory requirements and industry best practices. Specify the roles and responsibilities of the auditing and monitoring team, as well as the process for escalating identified issues.

5. **Resource Allocation:** Allocate sufficient resources, including personnel, technology, and financial resources, to support the auditing and monitoring efforts. Ensure that the auditing and monitoring team possesses the necessary expertise and skills to carry out their responsibilities effectively. Consider leveraging internal resources or engaging external experts as needed.

6. **Develop Audit and Monitoring Plans:** Create a comprehensive audit and monitoring plan that outlines the specific objectives, methodologies, and timelines for each audit or monitoring activity. Determine the frequency of audits and monitoring based on risk levels and regulatory requirements. Incorporate a mix of proactive and reactive audits, including both random and targeted audits.

7. **Data Collection and Analysis:** Establish processes for collecting and analyzing relevant data and information during audits and monitoring activities. Leverage technology solutions, data analytics tools, and automation to streamline data collection, enhance accuracy, and identify patterns or anomalies that may indicate non-compliance or potential risks.

8. **Reporting and Communication:** Develop a reporting framework to communicate audit and monitoring findings to appropriate stakeholders, such as senior management, compliance officers, and relevant departments. Ensure that the reports are comprehensive, clear, and actionable, highlighting areas of non-compliance, identified risks, and recommended corrective actions.

9. **Corrective Action and Follow-up:** Implement a process for tracking and managing corrective actions resulting from audit and monitoring findings. Establish mechanisms to ensure that identified non-compliance issues are addressed promptly, and appropriate remedial actions are taken. Monitor the implementation and effectiveness of corrective actions, and document the resolution process.

10. **Continuous Improvement:** Regularly evaluate and refine the auditing and monitoring framework based on feedback, changes in regulations, emerging risks, and internal lessons learned. Seek input from stakeholders, including auditors, compliance officers, and employees, to identify areas for improvement and enhance the effectiveness of the framework over time.

By following these steps, healthcare organizations can establish a robust auditing and monitoring framework that promotes regulatory compliance, identifies areas of non-compliance, and supports continuous improvement in adherence to applicable laws, regulations, and internal policies.

Conducting Internal Audits and Implementing Corrective Actions

Conducting internal audits and implementing corrective actions are critical steps in ensuring compliance and addressing non-compliance within healthcare organizations. Here's a guide on how to effectively conduct internal audits and implement corrective actions:

1. **Establish Audit Objectives:**

   Define the specific objectives of the internal audit, such as assessing compliance with regulations, identifying process inefficiencies, or evaluating the effectiveness of internal controls. Clearly articulate the scope, areas, and processes to be audited.

2. **Develop an Audit Plan:**

   Create a comprehensive audit plan that outlines the audit objectives, methodologies, timelines, and resource requirements. Consider using a risk-based approach to prioritize audits based on the level of risk and significance to compliance.

3. **Conduct Audit Fieldwork:**

   Perform the audit fieldwork by collecting and examining relevant data, documents, and records. Conduct interviews with employees and key stakeholders to gain insights and verify compliance practices. Apply appropriate auditing techniques, such as sampling, data analysis, and observation, to gather evidence.

4. **Assess Compliance and Identify Gaps:**

   Evaluate the audit findings against applicable laws, regulations, internal policies, and industry best practices. Identify areas of non-compliance, process inefficiencies, control weaknesses, or emerging risks. Document and communicate the audit findings accurately and objectively.

5. **Report Audit Findings:**

   Prepare a comprehensive audit report that includes a summary of the audit objectives, scope, methodologies, key findings, and recommendations. Clearly articulate the non-compliance issues, associated risks, and the potential impact on the organization. Provide practical and actionable recommendations for corrective actions.

6. **Implement Corrective Actions:**

Develop a corrective action plan based on the audit findings and recommendations. Assign responsibility to appropriate individuals or departments for addressing identified non-compliance issues. Establish specific timelines for implementing corrective actions and ensure they are realistic and achievable.

7. **Monitor Corrective Actions:**

Regularly monitor the progress of corrective actions to ensure timely and effective implementation. Track the status of each corrective action, document updates, and address any challenges or barriers. Communicate progress to relevant stakeholders and provide support as needed to facilitate successful implementation.

8. **Verify Effectiveness:**

Conduct follow-up audits or reviews to verify the effectiveness of implemented corrective actions. Assess whether the identified non-compliance issues have been resolved, processes have been improved, and controls have been strengthened. Document the results of the verification process for future reference.

9. **Documentation and Recordkeeping:**

Maintain thorough documentation of the entire audit process, including the audit plan, work papers, findings, recommendations, and implementation status of corrective actions. Ensure proper recordkeeping and retention of audit documentation in accordance with legal and organizational requirements.

10. **Continuous Improvement:**

Use the findings and lessons learned from internal audits to enhance compliance practices and promote a culture of continuous improvement. Consider incorporating audit feedback into policy updates, training programs, and process enhancements. Regularly review and update the internal audit plan to address emerging risks and changing compliance requirements.

By following these steps, healthcare organizations can conduct effective internal audits, identify non-compliance issues, and implement corrective actions to address those issues. This proactive approach helps ensure compliance with regulations, mitigate risks, and continuously improve compliance practices within the organization.

Leveraging Data Analytics for Compliance Monitoring and Risk Assessment

Leveraging data analytics for compliance monitoring and risk assessment can significantly enhance the effectiveness and efficiency of these processes in healthcare organizations. Here's how you can effectively utilize data analytics in compliance monitoring and risk assessment:

1. **Identify Relevant Data Sources:**

   Identify the key data sources that contain information relevant to compliance monitoring and risk assessment. This may include electronic health records (EHRs), billing and claims data, financial records, employee records, audit trails, and incident reports. Collaborate with IT and data management teams to ensure access to the necessary data.

2. **Define Compliance Indicators and Risk Factors:**

   Work with compliance officers and subject matter experts to identify compliance indicators and risk factors that can be monitored using data analytics. These can include patterns of billing errors, coding discrepancies, outlier claims, deviations from established protocols, employee behavior anomalies, or trends related to fraud and abuse.

3. **Develop Data Analytics Models:**

   Leverage data analytics tools and techniques to develop models and algorithms that can analyze large volumes of data and detect patterns, anomalies, or potential risks. This may involve using statistical analysis, machine learning algorithms, data visualization, or predictive modeling to identify patterns of non-compliance or assess the likelihood of potential risks.

4. **Data Cleaning and Preparation:**

   Ensure data integrity by cleaning and preparing the data for analysis. This includes removing duplicate records, handling missing data, standardizing data formats, and addressing data quality issues. Data cleansing processes should be performed to ensure accurate and reliable results.

5. **Analyze Compliance Data:**

Apply data analytics techniques to analyze compliance data and identify patterns or anomalies that may indicate non-compliance or potential risks. For example, analyze billing and claims data to detect coding errors, investigate patterns of overbilling, or identify unusual billing patterns. Use data visualization techniques to present the findings in a clear and understandable manner.

6. **Monitor Real-Time Data Streams:**

Implement real-time data monitoring to identify compliance issues as they occur. Set up automated data feeds and alerts to monitor key compliance indicators continuously. This allows for proactive identification of potential compliance breaches and immediate response to mitigate risks.

7. **Conduct Risk Assessments:**

Utilize data analytics to assess compliance risks by analyzing historical data, identifying trends, and applying predictive modeling to estimate future risks. This can help prioritize areas for focused monitoring and allocate resources effectively based on the level of risk.

8. **Establish Data Governance and Security:**

Ensure data governance and security measures are in place to protect sensitive and confidential information. Implement appropriate data access controls, encryption, and anonymization techniques to safeguard patient privacy and comply with data protection regulations.

9. **Continuous Monitoring and Improvement:**

Continuously monitor and refine the data analytics models, algorithms, and processes to improve accuracy and effectiveness. Regularly update the models to incorporate new compliance regulations, industry guidelines, or emerging risks. Analyze feedback and insights from data analytics to enhance compliance strategies, training programs, and internal controls.

10. **Collaboration and Communication:**

Collaborate with compliance officers, IT teams, data analysts, and other stakeholders to ensure effective use of data analytics for compliance monitoring and risk assessment. Communicate the findings, insights, and recommendations to relevant stakeholders, including senior management, compliance committees, and department heads.

By leveraging data analytics for compliance monitoring and risk assessment, healthcare organizations can gain valuable insights, detect non-compliance issues, and proactively address emerging risks. This data-driven approach enhances efficiency, accuracy, and effectiveness in identifying and mitigating compliance risks, ultimately strengthening the organization's overall compliance program.

Compliance in Medical Ethics and Research Misconduct

Compliance in medical ethics and research misconduct is essential to ensure the protection of human subjects, maintain the integrity of research, and uphold ethical standards in healthcare. Here's an overview of compliance considerations in medical ethics and research misconduct:

1. **Ethical Review and Approval:**

   Compliance in medical ethics begins with obtaining appropriate ethical review and approval for research involving human subjects. This typically involves submitting research proposals to an Institutional Review Board (IRB) or an Ethics Committee for evaluation of ethical implications, informed consent procedures, and protection of participants' rights and welfare.

2. **Informed Consent and Privacy Protection:**

   Compliance in medical ethics requires obtaining informed consent from research participants, ensuring they fully understand the purpose, risks, benefits, and procedures involved in the study. Privacy protection is also crucial to safeguard participants' personal information and medical records, adhering to applicable privacy laws and regulations such as HIPAA.

3. **Research Misconduct Policies and Procedures:**

   Healthcare organizations should have well-defined policies and procedures to address research misconduct, including fabrication, falsification, plagiarism, or other unethical practices. These policies should outline the process for reporting, investigating, and resolving allegations of research misconduct in a fair and unbiased manner.

4. **Training and Education:**

   Proper training and education on medical ethics and research misconduct are vital for researchers, healthcare professionals, and staff involved in research activities. Training programs should cover ethical principles, informed consent processes, privacy protection, and responsible conduct of research. Ongoing education helps ensure awareness of evolving ethical standards and compliance requirements.

5. **Monitoring and Auditing:**

Regular monitoring and auditing of research activities and protocols help detect any potential non-compliance with ethical guidelines and research misconduct. This can involve reviewing research documentation, participant consent forms, data collection procedures, and adherence to approved protocols. Monitoring helps identify deviations and take corrective actions promptly.

6. **Whistleblower Protections:**

Providing whistleblower protections is essential to encourage individuals to report research misconduct or ethical violations without fear of retaliation. Establish mechanisms for reporting concerns or misconduct anonymously and ensure appropriate investigations and protections for whistleblowers.

7. **Reporting and Investigation of Allegations:**

Promptly investigate any allegations of research misconduct or ethical violations through a fair and impartial process. Implement procedures to report and document findings, take appropriate disciplinary actions, and communicate outcomes to relevant parties, such as funding agencies, regulatory bodies, and affected participants.

8. **Collaboration and Adherence to Guidelines:**

Collaborate with professional associations, regulatory bodies, and research institutions to stay updated on ethical guidelines, codes of conduct, and best practices in medical ethics. Adherence to international standards, such as the Declaration of Helsinki and Good Clinical Practice (GCP) guidelines, helps ensure compliance with ethical requirements.

9. **Continuous Improvement and Training:**

Regularly review and update policies, procedures, and training programs based on lessons learned from research misconduct cases and emerging ethical issues. Foster a culture of continuous improvement, ethical awareness, and responsible research conduct through ongoing training and communication.

10. **Public Transparency and Accountability:**

Promote public transparency and accountability by publishing research findings, adhering to publication guidelines, and disclosing any conflicts of interest. Ensuring open communication and sharing research results responsibly contributes to maintaining the public's trust in research and ethical practices.

By emphasizing compliance in medical ethics and research misconduct, healthcare organizations can protect the rights and well-being of research participants, maintain the integrity of research outcomes, and uphold ethical standards in healthcare and scientific advancement.

Ethical Considerations in Medical Practice and Research

Ethical considerations play a critical role in both medical practice and research. They guide healthcare professionals and researchers in making decisions that prioritize the well-being and rights of patients and research participants. Here are key ethical considerations in medical practice and research (Figure 16.1):

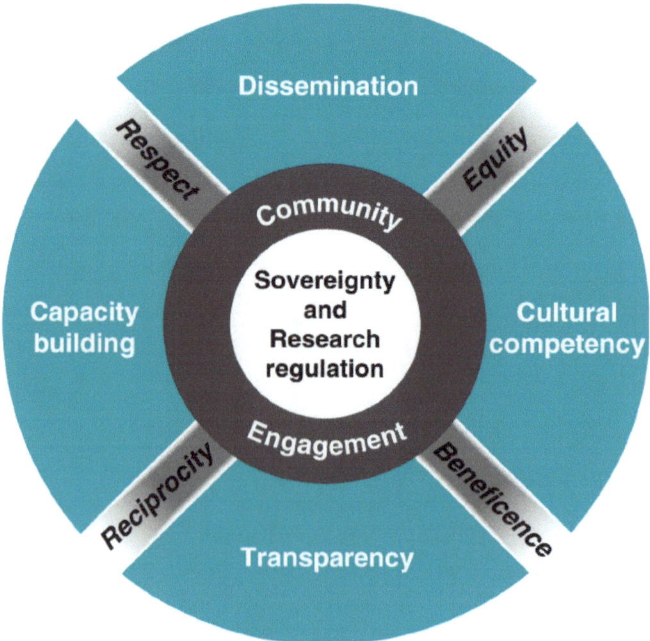

▼ **Figure 16.1:** Ethical Considerations in Medical Practice and Research

1. **Respect for Autonomy:**

   Respecting patient autonomy is fundamental to medical ethics. It involves honoring patients' right to make informed decisions about their own healthcare, including the right to consent to or refuse treatment. Healthcare professionals must provide patients with relevant information, ensure their understanding, and respect their choices.

2. **Beneficence and Non-maleficence:**

   The principles of beneficence and non-maleficence require healthcare professionals to act in the best interests of their patients, promoting their well-being and avoiding harm. This involves providing appropriate and effective treatments, minimizing risks, and considering the potential benefits and harms of interventions.

3. **Justice and Fairness:**

   Justice calls for fairness in the distribution of healthcare resources, access to medical services, and the allocation of research opportunities. Healthcare professionals and researchers must strive to ensure equitable access to healthcare and research participation, considering factors such as socioeconomic status, geographical location, and vulnerable populations.

4. **Informed Consent:**

   Obtaining informed consent is essential in both medical practice and research. Healthcare professionals must ensure that patients understand the nature, purpose, risks, and benefits of proposed treatments or interventions. In research, informed consent includes providing clear information about the study, potential risks, and the voluntary nature of participation.

5. **Privacy and Confidentiality:**

   Respecting patient privacy and maintaining confidentiality are crucial ethical considerations. Healthcare professionals must protect patients' personal health information and maintain confidentiality unless required by law or with the patient's consent. Researchers must also protect the privacy of research participants and handle data securely.

6. **Conflict of Interest:**

   Identifying and managing conflicts of interest is vital to maintain trust and integrity in medical practice and research. Healthcare professionals and researchers must disclose any financial or personal interests that could potentially bias their decision-making or compromise patient care or research integrity.

7. **Research Integrity and Rigor:**

In research, upholding integrity and rigor is essential. Researchers must adhere to ethical guidelines, accurately report methods and findings, avoid fabrication or falsification of data, and ensure the reproducibility of research. Transparent reporting of research methods, conflicts of interest, and funding sources is crucial for maintaining scientific integrity.

8. **Protection of Vulnerable Populations:**

Special attention must be given to the protection of vulnerable populations, including children, pregnant women, prisoners, and individuals with cognitive impairments. Extra safeguards are necessary to ensure their rights, well-being, and informed participation in medical practice and research.

9. **End-of-Life Care and Palliative Care:**

Ethical considerations in end-of-life care include respecting patients' wishes regarding life-sustaining treatments, providing comfort and dignity in the dying process, and involving patients and their families in decision-making. Palliative care focuses on alleviating suffering and enhancing the quality of life for patients with serious illnesses.

10. **Collaboration and Professionalism:**

Healthcare professionals and researchers should promote a collaborative and interdisciplinary approach, respecting the expertise and contributions of different professionals. Professionalism, including honesty, integrity, and respect for colleagues and patients, is essential in both medical practice and research.

By addressing these ethical considerations, healthcare professionals and researchers can ensure patient-centered care, protect research participants' rights, uphold integrity, and maintain public trust in medicine and research.

Compliance with Ethical Guidelines and Principles (Nuremberg Code, Belmont Report)

Compliance with ethical guidelines and principles is crucial in healthcare to ensure the protection of human subjects, respect for patient autonomy, and the ethical conduct of research. Two significant ethical frameworks that provide guidance in this regard are the Nuremberg Code and the Belmont Report:

1. **Nuremberg Code:**

   The Nuremberg Code emerged as a response to the unethical human experiments conducted during World War II. It emphasizes voluntary informed consent, stating that the subject's consent is essential in any research involving human subjects. Key principles of the Nuremberg Code include:

   - Informed Consent: Participants must give voluntary, informed, and uncoerced consent after receiving adequate information about the research.

   - Beneficence and Non-Maleficence: The well-being of participants must take precedence over the research objectives, and researchers should avoid causing harm.

   - Scientific Validity: Research should be based on sound scientific principles and experimentation, with a focus on minimizing unnecessary suffering or injury to participants.

2. **Belmont Report:**

   The Belmont Report, issued by the U.S. National Commission for the Protection of Human Subjects of Biomedical and Behavioral Research, provides ethical principles and guidelines for research involving human subjects. The report identifies three core principles that guide ethical research:

   - Respect for Persons: Researchers must respect the autonomy and dignity of individuals, ensuring informed consent and protecting vulnerable populations.

   - Beneficence: Researchers should maximize potential benefits while minimizing risks and harm to participants.

   - Justice: Fairness should govern the selection of research subjects, ensuring equal distribution of benefits and burdens.

Both the Nuremberg Code and the Belmont Report serve as essential ethical frameworks for research involving human subjects. Compliance with these guidelines and principles ensures the protection of participants' rights, promotes ethical research practices, and upholds the integrity of scientific inquiry.

In addition to the Nuremberg Code and the Belmont Report, other ethical guidelines and principles exist at the international and national levels. These include the Declaration of Helsinki, which provides ethical standards for medical research involving human subjects, and various guidelines issued by professional associations and regulatory bodies specific to different areas of medical practice and research.

Compliance with these ethical guidelines and principles is not only a legal and regulatory requirement but also an ethical obligation for healthcare professionals and researchers. It helps ensure the well-being and autonomy of patients and research participants, maintains public trust in the medical profession and research enterprise, and upholds the highest standards of ethical conduct in healthcare.

Addressing Research Misconduct and Ethical Violations

Addressing research misconduct and ethical violations is crucial to maintain the integrity of research and protect the well-being and rights of research participants. Here are key steps to address research misconduct and ethical violations effectively:

1. **Establish Policies and Procedures:** Develop clear policies and procedures that outline the process for reporting, investigating, and addressing research misconduct and ethical violations. These policies should define what constitutes misconduct, describe the reporting channels, and specify the responsibilities of key individuals or committees involved in the investigation process.

2. **Create a Reporting Mechanism:** Establish a confidential and anonymous reporting mechanism to encourage individuals to report suspected misconduct or ethical violations without fear of reprisal. Provide clear instructions on how to report concerns and ensure that all reports are taken seriously and investigated appropriately.

3. **Initiate a Thorough Investigation:** Once a report is received, initiate a thorough and impartial investigation. Assign a designated committee or an independent body to oversee the investigation process. This may involve reviewing relevant documents, conducting interviews with involved parties, and gathering evidence to substantiate the allegations.

4. **Ensure Due Process and Confidentiality:** Ensure that all individuals involved in the investigation are afforded due process rights, including the opportunity to provide their side of the story and respond to allegations. Maintain confidentiality throughout the investigation to protect the privacy and reputations of all parties involved.

5. **Collaboration with Relevant Authorities:** If the allegations involve potential violations of regulations or laws, collaborate with relevant authorities such as institutional compliance offices, funding agencies, regulatory bodies, or legal entities. Adhere to any legal reporting obligations and cooperate with external investigations as necessary.

6. **Determine Findings and Take Action:** Once the investigation is completed, determine the findings based on the evidence gathered. If research misconduct or ethical violations are substantiated, take appropriate disciplinary actions in accordance with established policies and applicable regulations. This may include corrective actions, sanctions, education or training, or termination of employment or research funding.

7. **Communicate Findings and Outcomes:** Communicate the findings and outcomes of the investigation to relevant parties, including affected individuals, institutional leadership, funding agencies, and regulatory bodies, as required. Maintain transparency and ensure that appropriate measures are implemented to prevent future occurrences of misconduct or ethical violations.

8. **Support Whistleblower Protections:** Provide support and protection for individuals who report research misconduct or ethical violations. Protect whistleblowers from retaliation and ensure a supportive environment where individuals feel safe to report concerns without fear of negative consequences.

9. **Implement Corrective Actions and Preventive Measures:** Implement corrective actions based on the investigation findings to address any identified deficiencies in research practices or institutional processes. Develop preventive measures, such as enhanced training programs, educational initiatives, and improved oversight mechanisms, to minimize the risk of future misconduct or ethical violations.

10. **Foster a Culture of Integrity:** Cultivate a culture of research integrity and ethical conduct by promoting responsible research practices, ethical training, and ongoing education. Establish regular ethics discussions,

training programs, and workshops to raise awareness and reinforce ethical standards among researchers and staff.

Addressing research misconduct and ethical violations requires a systematic and comprehensive approach. By implementing robust policies and procedures, fostering a culture of integrity, and taking prompt and appropriate actions when allegations arise, healthcare organizations can maintain the highest ethical standards in research and protect the welfare of research participants.

The Role of Institutional Review Boards (IRBs) in Promoting Compliance

Institutional Review Boards (IRBs) play a vital role in promoting compliance with ethical standards and protecting the rights and welfare of research participants. Here are the key roles and responsibilities of IRBs in promoting compliance:

1. **Ethical Review and Approval:**

   IRBs are responsible for reviewing research proposals involving human subjects to ensure that they adhere to ethical guidelines and regulations. They evaluate the research design, informed consent procedures, data collection methods, and potential risks and benefits to participants. The primary goal is to protect the rights, welfare, and privacy of research participants.

2. **Informed Consent Process:**

   IRBs review and assess the informed consent process to ensure that participants receive clear, understandable, and comprehensive information about the research study. They evaluate the adequacy of consent forms, participant information sheets, and any additional materials used to obtain informed consent. IRBs ensure that participants have the necessary information to make voluntary and informed decisions about their involvement in the research.

3. **Risk-Benefit Assessment:**

   IRBs carefully evaluate the potential risks and benefits of research studies. They assess whether the potential benefits of the research justify the risks involved. IRBs aim to minimize risks to participants and ensure that researchers have considered and addressed any potential harms or adverse effects associated with the study.

4. **Ongoing Monitoring and Review:**

   IRBs provide ongoing oversight of approved research studies to ensure that they continue to comply with ethical standards. They may conduct periodic reviews, inspections, or audits to verify compliance with approved protocols, participant safety, and ongoing informed consent. IRBs have the authority to suspend or terminate studies if non-compliance or ethical concerns are identified.

5. **Review of Amendments and Modifications:**

   IRBs review and approve any proposed amendments or modifications to research protocols. Researchers are required to seek IRB approval before implementing changes that may affect participant rights, safety, or the overall ethical conduct of the study. IRBs assess the potential impact of these modifications on participant welfare and compliance with ethical guidelines.

6. **Education and Training:**

   IRBs provide education and training to researchers, study coordinators, and other key personnel involved in research. They ensure that individuals conducting research are aware of and understand ethical guidelines, regulations, and the specific requirements of the IRB. Training programs help promote compliance and enhance ethical awareness among researchers.

7. **Compliance with Regulatory Requirements:**

   IRBs ensure compliance with local, national, and international regulations governing research involving human subjects. They monitor changes in regulations, guidelines, and ethical standards, and update their policies and procedures accordingly. IRBs serve as a resource for researchers, offering guidance on compliance and ethical considerations.

8. **Recordkeeping and Reporting:**

   IRBs maintain detailed records of all research protocols, reviews, and decisions. They ensure proper recordkeeping to document the ethical review process, correspondence, minutes of meetings, and any actions taken. IRBs may also report to regulatory authorities or funding agencies regarding compliance issues, adverse events, or serious breaches of ethical guidelines.

9. **Community Engagement and Public Trust:**

   IRBs engage with the community to raise awareness of research ethics and foster public trust. They may conduct outreach programs, participate in community forums, and respond to public concerns or inquiries related to research ethics. IRBs play a crucial role in ensuring that research is conducted in a manner that respects community values and safeguards the interests of research participants.

10. **Continuous Improvement:**

    IRBs strive for continuous improvement in their processes and practices. They actively seek feedback from researchers, participants, and other stakeholders to enhance the effectiveness and efficiency of the ethical review process. IRBs stay updated on emerging ethical issues, advancements in research methodologies, and evolving regulations to ensure ongoing compliance.

By fulfilling these roles and responsibilities, IRBs play a crucial role in promoting compliance with ethical standards, protecting research participants, and upholding the integrity of research. Their oversight and review processes help ensure that research studies are conducted in an ethical manner, with due consideration for participant rights, welfare, and informed consent. Through ongoing monitoring, education, and collaboration with researchers and the community, IRBs contribute to the promotion of ethical research practices and the maintenance of public trust in the research enterprise.

Compliance and Corporate Governance

Compliance and corporate governance are closely intertwined and mutually reinforcing concepts within organizations. Compliance refers to adherence to laws, regulations, policies, and ethical standards, while corporate governance encompasses the system of rules, practices, and processes that guide and control an organization's decision-making and behavior. Here's an overview of the relationship between compliance and corporate governance:

1. **Legal and Regulatory Compliance:**

   Compliance with laws and regulations is a fundamental aspect of corporate governance. Effective corporate governance frameworks ensure that organizations operate within the legal boundaries and comply with applicable regulations specific to their industry. Compliance programs and controls are put in place to monitor, assess, and mitigate legal and regulatory risks, ensuring the organization's actions align with legal requirements.

2. **Ethical Standards and Code of Conduct:**

   Corporate governance involves establishing and upholding ethical standards within an organization. This includes defining a code of conduct that outlines the expected behaviors and ethical principles for employees and stakeholders. Compliance with ethical standards is integral to maintaining the organization's reputation, fostering trust, and avoiding ethical violations.

3. **Risk Management and Internal Controls:**

   Corporate governance frameworks encompass robust risk management processes and internal controls. Compliance programs are designed to identify, assess, and mitigate risks that could lead to legal or ethical breaches. Internal controls ensure the effectiveness and efficiency of operations, safeguard assets, and promote compliance with laws and regulations.

4. **Board of Directors and Oversight:**

Corporate governance places significant emphasis on the role of the board of directors in overseeing organizational activities and ensuring compliance. The board has the responsibility to establish a culture of compliance, provide guidance on strategic decisions, and monitor management's compliance efforts. The board also appoints compliance officers or committees to oversee compliance activities.

5. **Transparency and Accountability:**

Effective corporate governance fosters transparency and accountability within an organization. Compliance with reporting and disclosure requirements ensures that stakeholders have access to accurate and reliable information about the organization's performance, risks, and compliance efforts. Transparency enhances trust and credibility, while accountability ensures that individuals and entities responsible for compliance are held answerable for their actions.

6. **Stakeholder Relationships and Engagement:**

Corporate governance involves managing relationships with various stakeholders, including shareholders, employees, customers, suppliers, and the wider community. Compliance with laws, regulations, and ethical standards is crucial to building and maintaining these relationships. Organizations with strong corporate governance practices demonstrate commitment to compliance, which can enhance stakeholder trust and loyalty.

7. **Enforcement and Consequences:**

Non-compliance with laws, regulations, and ethical standards can have severe consequences for organizations, including legal penalties, reputational damage, financial loss, and loss of public trust. Corporate governance frameworks ensure mechanisms for enforcement and accountability, allowing organizations to take appropriate actions against non-compliance, such as disciplinary measures, corrective actions, or internal investigations.

8. **Continuous Improvement and Adaptation:**

Corporate governance and compliance are not static concepts. They require continuous improvement, monitoring, and adaptation to evolving laws, regulations, and ethical standards. Organizations must regularly assess their governance structures, compliance programs, and internal controls to address emerging risks and changing compliance requirements.

By integrating compliance principles and practices into corporate governance frameworks, organizations can promote ethical conduct, mitigate risks, and ensure legal and regulatory compliance. A robust compliance program, overseen by effective corporate governance, enables organizations to operate with integrity, accountability, and transparency while fulfilling their obligations to stakeholders.

Integration of Compliance into Corporate Governance Structures

The integration of compliance into corporate governance structures is essential for organizations to effectively manage risks, ensure ethical behavior, and maintain legal and regulatory compliance. Here are key ways to integrate compliance into corporate governance structures:

1. **Board Oversight and Accountability:**

   Corporate governance frameworks should assign responsibility for compliance oversight to the board of directors. The board should establish a compliance committee or designate a specific board member with expertise in compliance to oversee and monitor the organization's compliance efforts. This ensures that compliance is given adequate attention, receives regular reporting, and is embedded in strategic decision-making.

2. **Compliance Policies and Code of Conduct:**

   Develop comprehensive compliance policies and a code of conduct that align with the organization's values, ethical standards, and legal requirements. These documents should be communicated to all employees, emphasizing the importance of compliance and setting clear expectations for behavior. Integrating compliance expectations into the code of conduct reinforces the organization's commitment to compliance and ethical practices.

3. **Risk Assessment and Management:**

   Integrate compliance considerations into the organization's overall risk assessment and management processes. Conduct regular risk assessments to identify compliance risks and prioritize them based on their potential impact.

This enables the organization to allocate resources effectively, implement controls, and establish mitigation strategies to address compliance risks.

4. **Compliance Reporting and Whistleblower Mechanisms:**

Establish mechanisms for employees and stakeholders to report compliance concerns and potential violations. Encourage a culture of open communication and provide confidential channels for reporting, such as a whistleblower hotline or an anonymous reporting system. Ensure that reports are promptly and thoroughly investigated, and appropriate actions are taken to address the issues raised.

5. **Compliance Training and Awareness:**

Provide regular compliance training programs to employees at all levels of the organization. Training should cover legal and regulatory requirements, the organization's compliance policies, and specific ethical considerations relevant to the industry. Reinforce compliance awareness through ongoing communication, newsletters, and internal campaigns to keep employees informed and engaged in compliance efforts.

6. **Compliance Performance Metrics and Reporting:**

Develop compliance performance metrics and establish reporting mechanisms to track and assess the effectiveness of compliance programs. Regularly monitor and measure compliance indicators, such as policy adherence, completion of training, incident reporting, and corrective actions. Reporting on compliance metrics to the board and senior management helps drive accountability and enables proactive decision-making.

7. **Integration with Internal Controls and Auditing:**

Integrate compliance considerations into the organization's internal controls framework and auditing processes. Ensure that compliance controls are embedded in operational processes to prevent and detect non-compliance. Regularly review and update internal controls to address emerging compliance risks and changes in regulations.

8. **Compliance as a Key Performance Indicator (KPI):**

Include compliance as a key performance indicator in the organization's overall performance measurement framework. This demonstrates the organization's commitment to compliance and reinforces its importance alongside other strategic objectives. Incorporate compliance metrics into performance evaluations and consider linking incentives to compliance achievements.

9. **Regular Compliance Assessments and Reviews:**

   Conduct periodic assessments and reviews of the organization's compliance program to evaluate its effectiveness and identify areas for improvement. Independent internal or external audits can provide an objective evaluation of compliance processes and controls. Use the findings and recommendations from these assessments to enhance the compliance program and align it with evolving best practices.

10. **Continuous Improvement and Adaptation:**

    Continuously monitor changes in laws, regulations, and industry standards to ensure the compliance program remains up to date. Stay informed about emerging compliance risks and adapt the compliance framework accordingly. Foster a culture of continuous improvement and learning, encouraging employees to provide feedback and suggestions for enhancing compliance practices.

By integrating compliance into corporate governance structures, organizations demonstrate their commitment to ethical behavior, risk management, and legal compliance. This integration fosters a culture of compliance, ensures accountability, and promotes sustainable business practices that align with regulatory requirements and stakeholder expectations. It strengthens the organization's reputation, builds trust with stakeholders, and mitigates compliance risks, ultimately contributing to the long-term success and sustainability of the organization.

Compliance Considerations for Board of Directors and Executive Management

Compliance considerations for the board of directors and executive management are essential to ensure effective oversight, accountability, and a strong culture of compliance within an organization. Here are key compliance considerations for the board of directors and executive management:

1. **Commitment to Compliance:** The board and executive management should demonstrate a strong commitment to compliance by prioritizing ethical behavior, legal compliance, and a culture of integrity throughout the organization. They should lead by example and communicate the importance of compliance in all aspects of the organization's operations.

2. **Compliance Oversight:** The board of directors should establish a clear governance structure that includes compliance oversight. This may involve

assigning compliance responsibilities to a dedicated committee or a specific board member with expertise in compliance. The board should receive regular compliance reports and updates to assess the effectiveness of the compliance program.

3. **Compliance Expertise:** The board and executive management should ensure that they have access to appropriate compliance expertise, either by having a director with compliance knowledge or by seeking external advice. This helps in understanding complex compliance issues, staying updated on regulatory changes, and making informed decisions regarding compliance-related matters.

4. **Risk Assessment and Management:** The board and executive management should be actively involved in the organization's risk assessment and management processes, including compliance risks. They should review and approve the organization's risk management strategies, ensuring that compliance risks are identified, assessed, and mitigated effectively.

5. **Compliance Policies and Procedures:** The board, in collaboration with executive management, should review and approve comprehensive compliance policies and procedures that align with legal and regulatory requirements. These policies should clearly articulate the organization's commitment to compliance, define expected behaviors, and provide guidance for employees to adhere to applicable laws and regulations.

6. **Communication and Training:** The board and executive management should emphasize the importance of compliance through regular communication channels. They should ensure that employees receive adequate training on compliance policies, procedures, and legal requirements. Communication should also address ethical standards, reporting mechanisms, and the consequences of non-compliance.

7. **Monitoring and Auditing:** The board and executive management should oversee the monitoring and auditing of the organization's compliance program. This includes reviewing compliance reports, internal audit findings, and external audit results. They should ensure that any identified compliance issues are addressed promptly and that appropriate corrective actions are implemented.

8. **Whistleblower Protections:** The board and executive management should establish and promote mechanisms for employees to report compliance concerns, such as a whistleblower hotline or anonymous reporting channels.

They should ensure that employees are aware of these mechanisms and that reports are promptly and thoroughly investigated.

9. **Ethics and Integrity:** The board and executive management should foster a culture of ethics and integrity throughout the organization. They should set the tone at the top by demonstrating ethical behavior and emphasizing the importance of integrity in all business dealings. This includes promoting transparency, accountability, and the responsible use of resources.

10. **Compliance Reporting and Accountability:** The board and executive management should ensure that they receive regular compliance reports and updates. They should review the organization's compliance performance, assess any compliance-related issues, and hold management accountable for maintaining a robust compliance program. This includes reviewing compliance metrics, key performance indicators, and taking appropriate action based on the findings.

By actively addressing these compliance considerations, the board of directors and executive management play a crucial role in fostering a culture of compliance, ensuring effective compliance oversight, and embedding compliance into the organization's governance structures. Their commitment to compliance sets the tone for the entire organization and helps establish a strong foundation for ethical behavior and legal compliance.

Transparency and Accountability in Compliance Reporting

Transparency and accountability in compliance reporting are crucial to ensure the effectiveness of compliance programs, maintain stakeholder trust, and demonstrate an organization's commitment to ethical behavior and legal compliance. Here are key considerations for promoting transparency and accountability in compliance reporting:

1. **Clear Reporting Framework:** Establish a clear reporting framework that outlines the requirements, expectations, and processes for compliance reporting. Clearly define the types of information to be reported, the frequency of reporting, and the channels through which reports should be submitted.

2. **Comprehensive Reporting Content:** Ensure that compliance reports provide comprehensive and accurate information about the organization's

compliance efforts. This includes reporting on compliance activities, key metrics, and any identified compliance issues or incidents. Reports should also highlight the organization's response to non-compliance and progress in addressing identified risks.

3. **Timeliness and Regularity:** Compliance reports should be timely and provided on a regular basis as defined in the reporting framework. This allows stakeholders to stay informed about the organization's compliance status and progress. Adhering to reporting timelines demonstrates the organization's commitment to transparency and accountability.

4. **Accuracy and Reliability:** Ensure that compliance reports are accurate, reliable, and based on verified data and information. Reports should undergo appropriate validation and verification processes to maintain their credibility. Proper documentation and recordkeeping are essential to support the accuracy and reliability of reported compliance information.

5. **Stakeholder Engagement:** Engage with relevant stakeholders to understand their expectations and information needs regarding compliance reporting. Seek feedback from stakeholders on the effectiveness and usefulness of the reports. Encourage stakeholder participation and involvement in the compliance reporting process to enhance transparency and accountability.

6. **Key Performance Indicators (KPIs):** Include relevant KPIs in compliance reporting to measure and demonstrate progress towards compliance objectives. KPIs should be aligned with the organization's compliance goals, such as policy adherence rates, training completion rates, incident response times, and corrective action implementation rates. Regularly assess and report on these KPIs to track performance and improvement.

7. **Root Cause Analysis and Corrective Actions:** Include information on the root causes of identified compliance issues and the corresponding corrective actions taken or planned. Describe the steps taken to address non-compliance, remediate the underlying causes, and prevent future occurrences. This demonstrates the organization's commitment to continuous improvement and learning from compliance incidents.

8. **Independent Review and Assurance:** Consider engaging external parties, such as auditors or consultants, to provide independent review and assurance of compliance reporting. External review helps validate the accuracy and reliability of the reports, enhancing their credibility and reinforcing the organization's commitment to transparency.

9. **Compliance Program Evaluation:** Include an assessment of the overall effectiveness of the compliance program in the reporting. Evaluate the compliance program against established objectives, performance metrics, and regulatory requirements. Identify areas for improvement and report on actions taken to strengthen the compliance program.

10. **Executive Management and Board Oversight:** Ensure that executive management and the board of directors are actively involved in compliance reporting. Provide regular updates to management and the board on compliance activities, issues, and trends. Executive management and the board should review and discuss compliance reports, ask relevant questions, and provide guidance and support to enhance transparency and accountability.

By incorporating these considerations into compliance reporting practices, organizations can promote transparency and accountability throughout their compliance programs. Transparent reporting enhances stakeholder confidence, supports informed decision-making, and fosters a culture of integrity and responsibility. It also enables organizations to identify areas for improvement, implement corrective actions, and continually enhance their compliance efforts.

The Role of Compliance in Promoting Organizational Integrity and Ethics

Compliance plays a vital role in promoting organizational integrity and ethics. It provides a framework for organizations to uphold ethical standards, maintain legal and regulatory compliance, and foster a culture of integrity throughout all levels of the organization. Here are the key ways in which compliance promotes organizational integrity and ethics:

1. **Setting Ethical Standards:** Compliance programs establish and communicate ethical standards that guide employee behavior and decision-making. They define the organization's values, code of conduct, and expectations for ethical behavior, creating a foundation for a culture of integrity.

2. **Legal and Regulatory Compliance:** Compliance ensures that organizations operate within the bounds of applicable laws, regulations, and industry standards. By adhering to legal requirements, organizations demonstrate their commitment to ethical business practices, avoiding legal pitfalls, and protecting the interests of stakeholders.

3. **Preventing Misconduct and Unethical Behavior:** Compliance programs are designed to prevent misconduct and unethical behavior within an organization. They provide guidelines, policies, and procedures that help employees understand what is expected of them and the consequences of non-compliance. This serves as a deterrent and promotes ethical decision-making.

4. **Ethical Decision-Making:** Compliance programs often include ethical decision-making frameworks that help employees navigate complex situations and make ethical choices. By promoting ethical decision-making processes, compliance supports integrity and fosters a culture where ethical behavior is valued and rewarded.

5. **Training and Education:** Compliance programs provide training and educational initiatives that raise awareness about ethical standards, legal requirements, and best practices. These initiatives help employees understand their ethical responsibilities and provide guidance on handling ethical dilemmas, promoting a culture of ethics and integrity.

6. **Reporting and Whistleblower Protections:** Compliance programs establish reporting mechanisms, such as anonymous hotlines or dedicated channels, to encourage employees to report unethical behavior or compliance concerns. Whistleblower protections ensure that employees can come forward without fear of retaliation, enabling the organization to address and rectify ethical issues promptly.

7. **Transparency and Accountability:** Compliance promotes transparency by requiring organizations to document and disclose their compliance efforts. Regular reporting on compliance activities, training completion rates, incident response, and corrective actions fosters accountability and demonstrates the organization's commitment to integrity.

8. **Third-Party Relationships:** Compliance programs extend to managing relationships with third parties, such as suppliers, contractors, and business partners. Organizations require their partners to adhere to ethical and compliance standards, ensuring that they conduct business in an ethical and responsible manner.

9. **Auditing and Monitoring:** Compliance programs incorporate auditing and monitoring processes to assess adherence to ethical standards and regulatory requirements. Regular internal and external audits help identify potential compliance gaps, monitor controls, and provide insights for improvement.

10. **Organizational Reputation and Trust:** Organizations with strong compliance programs and a commitment to ethics and integrity build a positive reputation and foster trust among stakeholders. This enhances the organization's standing in the marketplace, attracts top talent, and cultivates long-term relationships with customers, employees, investors, and the community.

By integrating compliance practices and ethical considerations into the fabric of the organization, compliance programs promote organizational integrity, instill ethical values, and contribute to a positive corporate culture. They create a framework where employees understand their ethical responsibilities, are empowered to make ethical decisions, and are held accountable for their actions. Ultimately, compliance programs play a pivotal role in shaping an organization's ethical identity and fostering a culture of integrity throughout the entire organization.

Compliance in Global Healthcare Operations

Compliance in global healthcare operations is essential to ensure that healthcare organizations adhere to applicable laws, regulations, and ethical standards in their international activities. As healthcare organizations expand their operations globally, they face unique compliance challenges due to varying regulatory environments, cultural differences, and diverse healthcare systems. Here are key considerations for compliance in global healthcare operations:

1. **Understanding International Regulations:** Healthcare organizations must have a thorough understanding of the regulatory frameworks in each country where they operate. This includes regulations related to licensing, healthcare delivery, data privacy and protection, drug and device approvals, clinical trials, and professional qualifications. Compliance teams should stay updated on changes in regulations and ensure that local compliance requirements are met.

2. **Adapting to Cultural and Ethical Differences:** Compliance programs should consider cultural and ethical differences across different regions and countries. Organizations must navigate local norms, customs, and legal expectations to ensure that their operations align with local ethical standards. This may involve adapting policies, training programs, and compliance practices to address cultural nuances and promote ethical behavior.

3. **Data Privacy and Security Compliance:** Healthcare organizations operating globally must comply with various data privacy and security regulations, such as the General Data Protection Regulation (GDPR) in the European Union. They must implement measures to protect patient data, including appropriate consent mechanisms, data transfer agreements, and data breach notification processes, while ensuring compliance with local data protection laws.

4. **Anti-Corruption and Bribery Laws:** Healthcare organizations must comply with anti-corruption and bribery laws, such as the U.S. Foreign Corrupt

Practices Act (FCPA) and the UK Bribery Act. They should establish policies and procedures to prevent bribery and corruption in international business dealings and provide training to employees on these laws.

5. **Vendor and Supply Chain Compliance:** Global healthcare operations involve engaging with vendors, suppliers, and third-party partners. Compliance programs should include due diligence processes to assess the compliance and integrity of these entities. Contracts and agreements should incorporate compliance expectations and require adherence to applicable laws and regulations.

6. **Managing International Clinical Trials:** Conducting international clinical trials requires compliance with local regulations, ethical guidelines, and informed consent requirements. Compliance teams must navigate different regulatory approval processes, monitor trial activities, and ensure adherence to international standards for trial conduct and participant protection.

7. **Cross-Border Licensing and Credentialing:** Healthcare professionals working in global operations may require licensing or credentialing in multiple jurisdictions. Compliance teams must understand the licensing requirements and ensure that healthcare professionals meet the necessary qualifications and comply with local regulations. This includes verifying credentials, monitoring license expiration dates, and managing the process for obtaining licenses in new jurisdictions.

8. **Training and Awareness:** Effective training and awareness programs are essential for global compliance. Healthcare organizations should provide training to employees working in international operations on applicable laws, regulations, cultural differences, and ethical considerations. This helps foster a compliance culture and ensures that employees understand their responsibilities and the potential risks associated with non-compliance.

9. **Centralized Compliance Oversight:** Establishing centralized compliance oversight is crucial for effective global compliance management. This involves coordinating compliance efforts across different regions, sharing best practices, and establishing consistent compliance standards and reporting mechanisms. Centralized oversight helps ensure that compliance programs are aligned with organizational goals and that risks are appropriately managed.

10. **Collaboration with Local Partners:** Engaging with local partners, such as healthcare providers, government agencies, and community organizations,

is essential for compliance in global healthcare operations. Collaborating with local stakeholders helps navigate the regulatory landscape, understand local expectations, and establish relationships based on trust and mutual compliance objectives.

By addressing these considerations, healthcare organizations can develop robust compliance programs that are tailored to the unique challenges of global healthcare operations. This promotes ethical practices, mitigates compliance risks, and ensures that healthcare services are delivered with integrity and in compliance with applicable laws and regulations and the highest standards of patient care. Compliance in global healthcare operations is an ongoing effort that requires organizations to stay informed, adaptable, and committed to ethical conduct across borders.

International Regulations and Standards for Healthcare Compliance

In the realm of healthcare compliance, several international regulations and standards play a significant role in guiding organizations' practices and ensuring consistency across borders. Here are some key international regulations and standards for healthcare compliance:

1. **World Health Organization (WHO) Guidelines:** The WHO develops guidelines and frameworks to promote health and healthcare globally. These guidelines cover various aspects of healthcare, including patient safety, quality improvement, infection prevention and control, ethical considerations, and health system strengthening.

2. **International Organization for Standardization (ISO) Standards:** ISO develops globally recognized standards that help organizations establish and maintain effective compliance and quality management systems. Relevant ISO standards for healthcare compliance include ISO 9001 (Quality Management Systems), ISO 27001 (Information Security Management Systems), and ISO 31000 (Risk Management).

3. **Good Clinical Practice (GCP):** GCP is an international ethical and scientific quality standard for designing, conducting, recording, and reporting clinical trials involving human subjects. It ensures the protection of participants' rights, safety, and well-being, and the reliability and integrity of trial data.

4. **International Council for Harmonization of Technical Requirements for Pharmaceuticals for Human Use (ICH):** The ICH develops guidelines for the pharmaceutical industry to promote the safety, efficacy, and quality of medicinal products. These guidelines cover various areas, including clinical trials, quality management systems, drug registration, and post-marketing surveillance.

5. **Data Privacy and Protection Laws:** Data privacy and protection laws, such as the European Union's General Data Protection Regulation (GDPR), govern the handling of personal data. These laws establish rights for individuals and impose obligations on organizations to protect personal data, obtain consent for its use, and implement appropriate security measures.

6. **Anti-Corruption and Anti-Bribery Laws:** International anti-corruption laws, such as the U.S. Foreign Corrupt Practices Act (FCPA) and the UK Bribery Act, prohibit bribery and corrupt practices in business transactions. These laws apply to healthcare organizations operating globally and require implementing measures to prevent corruption and bribery.

7. **Health Insurance Portability and Accountability Act (HIPAA):** Although primarily applicable to the United States, HIPAA's privacy and security rules have influenced data protection practices globally. Organizations that handle personal health information often adopt similar principles to safeguard patient privacy and ensure the secure exchange of healthcare data.

8. **Medical Device Regulations:** Various countries and regions have specific regulations for medical devices, such as the European Union's Medical Device Regulation (EU MDR) and the U.S. Food and Drug Administration's (FDA) regulations. These regulations govern the design, manufacturing, marketing, and post-market surveillance of medical devices.

9. **Anti-Money Laundering (AML) Regulations:** AML regulations aim to prevent the use of healthcare organizations for money laundering or financing of illegal activities. They require organizations to implement robust compliance programs, perform due diligence on customers and business partners, and report suspicious activities.

10. **National and Local Regulations:** Each country has its own healthcare regulations and requirements that organizations must comply with. These may include licensing and accreditation requirements, healthcare

professional qualifications, advertising and marketing regulations, and pricing and reimbursement guidelines.

Compliance with international regulations and standards is essential for healthcare organizations operating on a global scale. It helps ensure consistency, patient safety, data protection, ethical conduct, and adherence to best practices across borders. Organizations should stay informed about relevant regulations, continuously assess their compliance programs, and adapt their practices to meet international standards while also addressing local requirements in each jurisdiction of operation.

Navigating Cultural and Legal Differences in Global Compliance

Navigating cultural and legal differences is a crucial aspect of global compliance. Healthcare organizations operating in multiple countries must be sensitive to the cultural nuances and legal frameworks of each jurisdiction to effectively implement compliance programs. Here are some considerations for navigating cultural and legal differences in global compliance:

1. **Cultural Intelligence and Sensitivity:** Develop cultural intelligence within the compliance team and across the organization. Understand the cultural norms, values, and expectations of the countries in which the organization operates. Respect cultural differences and adapt compliance practices accordingly, ensuring that they align with local values and customs.

2. **Local Legal Expertise:** Seek legal expertise and guidance from professionals who are knowledgeable about the specific legal frameworks of each jurisdiction. Engage local legal counsel to understand and comply with local laws, regulations, and compliance requirements. This helps mitigate legal risks and ensures that compliance efforts are tailored to the local legal landscape.

3. **Compliance Localization:** Customize compliance policies, procedures, and training materials to address local legal and cultural considerations. Adapt the organization's compliance program to align with local regulations and expectations. Translate compliance materials into local languages to ensure understanding and compliance by employees in different regions.

4. **Stakeholder Engagement:** Engage with local stakeholders, including employees, customers, regulators, and community representatives. Seek

their input, understand their perspectives, and involve them in compliance initiatives. Building relationships with local stakeholders helps foster trust, gain valuable insights, and navigate cultural and legal differences effectively.

5. **Ethical Leadership:** Promote ethical leadership at all levels of the organization, emphasizing the importance of ethical conduct and integrity across cultural contexts. Leaders should lead by example and demonstrate a commitment to compliance and ethical behavior, regardless of cultural differences.

6. **Training and Communication:** Develop comprehensive compliance training programs that address cultural and legal differences. Provide training to employees on local laws, regulations, and ethical expectations. Emphasize the organization's commitment to compliance and ethical conduct, ensuring that employees understand their roles and responsibilities.

7. **Compliance Champions and Local Compliance Officers:** Appoint local compliance champions or compliance officers in each jurisdiction to serve as points of contact and experts on local compliance matters. These individuals can bridge the gap between global compliance standards and local requirements, providing guidance and ensuring compliance within their respective regions.

8. **Monitoring and Auditing:** Implement monitoring and auditing processes to assess compliance across different jurisdictions. Conduct regular compliance audits, including country-specific assessments, to identify compliance gaps and address any cultural or legal differences. Ensure that audit processes are sensitive to local practices and requirements.

9. **Reporting and Whistleblower Mechanisms:** Establish reporting mechanisms that are culturally sensitive and accessible to employees in different regions. Ensure that reporting channels are available in local languages and provide protections for whistleblowers. Communicate the organization's commitment to addressing compliance concerns and taking appropriate action.

10. **Continuous Learning and Improvement:** Foster a culture of continuous learning and improvement in global compliance efforts. Encourage feedback from employees in different regions, learn from experiences, and adapt compliance practices accordingly. Regularly review and update compliance programs to address cultural and legal differences and emerging risks.

Navigating cultural and legal differences in global compliance requires organizations to be adaptive, culturally sensitive, and responsive to local regulations and expectations. By incorporating these considerations, healthcare organizations can navigate the complexities of global compliance more effectively and maintain ethical and compliant operations across borders.

Strategies for Managing Compliance across International Operations

Managing compliance across international operations requires a strategic approach to address the unique challenges posed by different jurisdictions, cultural differences, and regulatory frameworks. Here are some strategies for effectively managing compliance across international operations:

1. **Comprehensive Compliance Program:** Develop a comprehensive compliance program that addresses global and local compliance requirements. The program should include policies, procedures, and guidelines that reflect the organization's commitment to compliance and adherence to applicable laws and regulations in each jurisdiction of operation.

2. **Centralized Compliance Oversight:** Establish centralized oversight for compliance to ensure consistency and coordination across international operations. This centralization allows for the development and implementation of consistent compliance policies, training programs, reporting mechanisms, and monitoring activities.

3. **Country-Specific Compliance Assessment:** Conduct country-specific compliance assessments to understand the legal and regulatory requirements of each jurisdiction. Identify the key compliance risks and challenges specific to each country and develop tailored strategies to address them. Engage local compliance officers or consultants with expertise in the specific jurisdiction to provide guidance and support.

4. **Regular Compliance Training:** Provide regular compliance training to employees across international operations. The training should cover key compliance topics, such as legal requirements, ethical standards, cultural considerations, and specific regulations applicable in each country. Tailor the training content to address the unique compliance challenges of each jurisdiction.

5. **Clear Communication Channels:** Establish clear communication channels to facilitate the reporting of compliance concerns and ensure timely communication across international operations. Provide employees with multiple avenues to report compliance issues, including anonymous reporting mechanisms. Regularly communicate updates on compliance policies, changes in regulations, and best practices to enhance awareness and understanding.

6. **Collaboration with Local Partners:** Foster collaboration with local partners, such as healthcare providers, regulators, and industry associations, to gain insights into local compliance requirements and best practices. Engage in ongoing dialogue and share knowledge to ensure alignment with local regulations and promote a culture of compliance in the local context.

7. **Robust Due Diligence Processes:** Implement robust due diligence processes for third-party relationships, including vendors, suppliers, and business partners. Ensure that these entities comply with applicable laws, regulations, and ethical standards. Conduct regular assessments and audits to monitor the compliance performance of third parties.

8. **Regular Compliance Monitoring and Auditing:** Establish a program of regular compliance monitoring and auditing across international operations. This includes conducting internal audits, risk assessments, and compliance reviews to identify areas of non-compliance and implement corrective actions. Monitor compliance metrics and key performance indicators to track compliance effectiveness.

9. **Continuous Regulatory Monitoring:** Stay abreast of regulatory changes and updates in each jurisdiction of operation. Monitor developments in laws, regulations, and industry guidelines to ensure compliance. Engage with local legal counsel and regulatory bodies to understand and interpret the evolving regulatory landscape.

10. **Ethical Tone at the Top:** Foster an ethical tone at the top by promoting a strong ethical culture within the organization. Ensure that leaders and executives set a positive example by consistently demonstrating ethical behavior and a commitment to compliance. This sends a clear message that compliance is a top priority across international operations.

By implementing these strategies, healthcare organizations can effectively manage compliance across international operations. They can navigate the complexities of different jurisdictions, cultural differences, and regulatory frameworks while maintaining a strong culture of compliance and ethical conduct throughout the organization.

Addressing Corruption Risks and Implementing Anti-bribery Measures

Addressing corruption risks and implementing anti-bribery measures is crucial for healthcare organizations operating in international contexts. Corruption can undermine ethical practices, compromise patient safety, and damage an organization's reputation. Here are strategies to address corruption risks and implement effective anti-bribery measures:

1. **Clear Anti-Bribery Policy:** Develop and communicate a clear anti-bribery policy that explicitly prohibits bribery, corruption, and unethical practices. The policy should outline the organization's commitment to integrity and compliance with applicable laws and regulations. Ensure that the policy is widely disseminated and accessible to all employees, contractors, and business partners.

2. **Conduct Risk Assessment:** Conduct a comprehensive risk assessment to identify corruption risks specific to the countries and regions in which the organization operates. Assess the potential risks associated with interactions with government officials, regulatory agencies, and other stakeholders. This assessment helps prioritize anti-bribery measures and allocate resources effectively.

3. **Due Diligence on Third Parties:** Implement robust due diligence procedures for assessing the integrity and compliance record of third parties, including vendors, suppliers, agents, consultants, and business partners. Evaluate their anti-bribery policies, ethical standards, and compliance practices before entering into any agreements or partnerships.

4. **Implement Anti-Bribery Controls:** Establish internal controls and procedures to prevent bribery and corruption. This includes implementing segregation of duties, financial controls, and approval processes to ensure transparency and accountability. Implement controls to monitor and detect suspicious transactions and facilitate reporting of potential bribery incidents.

5. **Training and Awareness:** Provide regular training programs to educate employees and relevant stakeholders about the risks of bribery and corruption. Training should cover the organization's anti-bribery policies,

local laws and regulations, red flags, and reporting mechanisms. Foster a culture of integrity by promoting ethical behavior and encouraging employees to report any suspected corrupt practices.

6. **Whistleblower Protection:** Establish a robust and confidential whistleblowing mechanism that allows employees and stakeholders to report suspected bribery or corruption without fear of retaliation. Ensure that whistleblower protection policies are in place and communicated effectively. Investigate and respond promptly to reported incidents.

7. **Monitoring and Auditing:** Conduct regular monitoring and auditing of anti-bribery measures to assess their effectiveness and identify potential weaknesses or gaps. This includes reviewing financial transactions, contracts, and relationships with high-risk entities. Independent audits can provide an objective assessment of the organization's compliance with anti-bribery policies.

8. **Reporting and Investigation Protocols:** Develop clear protocols for reporting and investigating alleged cases of bribery or corruption. Establish a dedicated internal reporting mechanism, investigate reported incidents promptly and impartially, and take appropriate disciplinary or legal action when warranted. Cooperate with relevant authorities and regulatory bodies as necessary.

9. **Collaboration with Industry and Government:** Engage in industry collaborations and share best practices to combat bribery and corruption. Collaborate with government agencies and industry associations to stay informed about new regulations, participate in anti-corruption initiatives, and contribute to industry-wide efforts to address corruption risks.

10. **Continuous Improvement:** Foster a culture of continuous improvement by regularly reviewing and enhancing anti-bribery measures. Stay updated on emerging trends, legal developments, and best practices in anti-corruption efforts. Conduct periodic reviews of policies, procedures, and training programs to ensure their relevance and effectiveness.

By implementing these strategies, healthcare organizations can proactively address corruption risks, promote ethical behavior, and safeguard their operations against bribery and corruption. Compliance with anti-bribery measures demonstrates a commitment to ethical business practices and helps protect the organization's reputation and integrity in international healthcare operations.

Compliance in Healthcare Mergers and Acquisitions

Compliance in healthcare mergers and acquisitions (M&A) is a critical consideration to ensure that the combined entity adheres to applicable laws, regulations, and ethical standards. M&A activities in the healthcare industry present unique compliance challenges due to the complex regulatory environment, potential for increased market power, and the need to protect patient safety and privacy. Here are key factors to consider for compliance in healthcare M&A:

1. **Due Diligence:** Conduct comprehensive due diligence on the target organization to assess its compliance program, regulatory history, and potential risks. Evaluate the target's compliance with laws and regulations, including healthcare-specific regulations such as HIPAA, Stark Law, and Anti-Kickback Statute. Identify any compliance issues or liabilities that may impact the transaction and develop a plan to address them.

2. **Regulatory Approvals:** Determine the regulatory approvals required for the M&A transaction, such as antitrust clearances, change of ownership filings, and licensing requirements. Ensure compliance with applicable laws and regulations governing mergers and acquisitions in the healthcare sector. Engage with regulatory authorities early in the process to address any concerns and obtain necessary approvals.

3. **Integration Planning:** Develop a comprehensive integration plan that includes compliance considerations. Assess the compliance programs of both entities and identify areas of alignment and potential gaps. Develop a roadmap for integrating compliance policies, procedures, and systems to ensure consistent and effective compliance across the combined organization.

4. **Patient Privacy and Data Protection:** Address patient privacy and data protection during the M&A process. Evaluate the data privacy and security practices of both organizations and develop a plan to align them.

Ensure compliance with data protection laws, such as HIPAA or GDPR, and implement measures to protect patient information throughout the integration process.

5. **Cultural Integration:** Recognize and address cultural differences in compliance practices between the acquiring and target organizations. Develop a strategy to harmonize compliance cultures and create a unified compliance framework. Foster open communication, provide training and support to employees, and ensure that compliance expectations are clearly communicated and understood.

6. **Compliance Program Enhancement:** Leverage the strengths of both organizations' compliance programs to enhance the overall compliance framework of the combined entity. Identify best practices, policies, and procedures from each organization and integrate them into a unified compliance program. Ensure that the compliance program addresses the specific risks and challenges associated with the M&A transaction.

7. **Employee Education and Training:** Provide comprehensive education and training to employees on the compliance expectations of the combined entity. This includes educating employees on new compliance policies, procedures, and codes of conduct resulting from the M&A. Train employees on any changes in laws and regulations that may affect their roles and responsibilities.

8. **Ongoing Monitoring and Auditing:** Establish ongoing monitoring and auditing processes to assess compliance effectiveness post-M&A. Conduct regular compliance audits and risk assessments to identify and mitigate potential compliance risks. Monitor compliance metrics and key performance indicators to ensure ongoing compliance with applicable laws and regulations.

9. **Post-Merger Compliance Integration:** Monitor the progress of compliance integration efforts post-merger and address any challenges or issues that arise. Continuously evaluate the effectiveness of the compliance program and make necessary adjustments to ensure ongoing compliance in the combined entity.

10. **Reporting and Whistleblower Protection:** Maintain robust reporting mechanisms and whistleblower protection policies to encourage employees to report compliance concerns. Establish a culture that encourages openness and transparency in reporting potential violations. Promptly investigate reported incidents and take appropriate remedial actions when necessary.

By considering these factors and implementing a well-planned compliance strategy, healthcare organizations can navigate the compliance challenges associated with M&A transactions and ensure a smooth integration while maintaining compliance with applicable laws, regulations, and ethical standards. Compliance should be a key focus throughout the M&A process to protect the organization's reputation, patient safety, and overall business integrity.

Compliance Considerations during Mergers, Acquisitions, and Partnerships

Compliance considerations during mergers, acquisitions, and partnerships are crucial to ensure that all parties involved adhere to applicable laws, regulations, and ethical standards. Here are some key compliance considerations to keep in mind during these transactions:

1. **Due Diligence:** Conduct thorough due diligence on the target company or partner to assess their compliance history, regulatory standing, and potential risks. Identify any compliance issues or liabilities that may impact the transaction and develop a plan to address them.

2. **Regulatory Compliance:** Ensure compliance with relevant regulatory requirements governing mergers, acquisitions, and partnerships in the specific industry or sector. This may include obtaining necessary approvals from regulatory authorities and complying with antitrust laws, change of ownership filings, licensing requirements, and other industry-specific regulations.

3. **Contractual Agreements:** Clearly define compliance expectations in contractual agreements between the parties involved. Include provisions that outline responsibilities for compliance, adherence to laws and regulations, and consequences for non-compliance. Specify mechanisms for monitoring and auditing compliance and dispute resolution processes.

4. **Data Privacy and Security:** Address data privacy and security considerations, particularly when sharing sensitive information during the transaction. Develop protocols to protect the privacy and security of personal and confidential data, ensuring compliance with applicable data protection laws and regulations.

5. **Anti-Corruption and Anti-Bribery Measures:** Implement robust anti-corruption and anti-bribery measures to prevent illegal practices. Ensure

that all parties involved understand and adhere to anti-corruption laws and regulations, such as the U.S. Foreign Corrupt Practices Act (FCPA) and the UK Bribery Act. Conduct appropriate due diligence on partners and third parties to mitigate corruption risks.

6. **Integration Planning:** Develop an integration plan that includes compliance considerations. Assess the compliance programs of the merging or partnering entities and identify areas of alignment and potential gaps. Develop a roadmap for integrating compliance policies, procedures, and systems to ensure consistent and effective compliance across the combined organization.

7. **Employee Education and Training:** Provide comprehensive compliance education and training to employees of the merging or partnering entities. Ensure that employees understand their roles and responsibilities in the new organizational structure, including compliance obligations and any changes resulting from the transaction. Reinforce the importance of ethical conduct and compliance with laws and regulations.

8. **Internal Controls and Monitoring:** Establish robust internal controls and monitoring mechanisms to ensure ongoing compliance. Implement processes to identify, assess, and mitigate compliance risks, including regular monitoring and auditing of compliance activities. Monitor compliance metrics and key performance indicators to track and evaluate compliance performance.

9. **Whistleblower Protection:** Maintain effective whistleblower protection mechanisms that encourage employees to report compliance concerns without fear of retaliation. Establish clear reporting channels and procedures for addressing whistleblower complaints. Promptly investigate reported incidents and take appropriate remedial actions when necessary.

10. **Post-Transaction Compliance Integration:** Monitor and evaluate the progress of compliance integration efforts post-transaction. Continuously assess the effectiveness of the compliance program and make necessary adjustments to ensure ongoing compliance in the merged or partnered entity. Regularly review and update compliance policies and procedures to reflect changes in laws and regulations.

By considering these compliance considerations throughout the merger, acquisition, or partnership process, organizations can better manage compliance risks, maintain integrity, and ensure adherence to laws, regulations, and ethical standards.

Compliance should be an integral part of the transaction planning and integration process to protect the reputation and long-term success of the organization.

Due Diligence and Assessing Compliance Risks in Transactions

Due diligence and assessing compliance risks are critical steps in transactions to ensure that potential risks and liabilities are identified and addressed. Here are key considerations for due diligence and assessing compliance risks in transactions:

1. **Compliance Review:** Conduct a comprehensive review of the target company or partner's compliance program, policies, and practices. Assess the effectiveness of their compliance program in mitigating risks and ensuring adherence to applicable laws, regulations, and industry standards. Review compliance-related documentation, including policies, procedures, training records, incident reports, and audit findings.

2. **Legal and Regulatory Compliance:** Evaluate the target company's compliance with relevant laws and regulations in its industry and jurisdiction. Identify any violations, penalties, or ongoing investigations. Assess compliance with specific regulations such as data protection, healthcare regulations, environmental regulations, anti-corruption laws, and employment laws.

3. **Contractual Obligations:** Review contractual agreements, licenses, permits, and certifications to ensure compliance with contractual obligations. Identify any potential breaches or non-compliance with contractual terms, including obligations related to intellectual property, confidentiality, quality standards, and regulatory compliance.

4. **Risk Assessment:** Conduct a risk assessment to identify compliance risks associated with the transaction. Evaluate risks related to legal, financial, operational, reputational, and strategic aspects of the target company or partner. Consider the impact of non-compliance on the transaction and the potential costs and consequences of identified risks.

5. **Compliance Culture:** Assess the target company or partner's compliance culture and commitment to ethical conduct. Evaluate their tone at the top, leadership commitment to compliance, and overall organizational culture. Consider the effectiveness of their compliance training,

communication, and reporting mechanisms in promoting a culture of compliance.

6. **Third-Party Relationships:** Evaluate the target company's relationships with third parties, including suppliers, contractors, agents, and distributors. Assess the due diligence conducted on third parties and their compliance with applicable laws and regulations. Determine any potential risks arising from these relationships, such as corruption, bribery, or inadequate data protection practices.

7. **Data Privacy and Security:** Assess the target company's data privacy and security practices, including their compliance with applicable data protection laws and regulations. Review data handling procedures, security measures, and any past data breaches or incidents. Evaluate the adequacy of data protection policies, consent mechanisms, and data transfer practices.

8. **Financial Controls:** Review financial records, internal controls, and compliance with accounting standards. Assess the target company's financial reporting practices, tax compliance, and anti-money laundering measures. Identify any irregularities, financial risks, or potential fraud-related issues.

9. **Environmental and Health Safety Compliance:** Evaluate the target company's compliance with environmental regulations and health and safety standards. Assess their practices related to waste management, pollution control, workplace safety, and employee health protection. Identify any past violations or liabilities related to environmental or safety compliance.

10. **Legal and Regulatory Changes:** Consider the potential impact of upcoming or recent legal and regulatory changes on the target company or partner's compliance obligations. Assess their readiness to adapt to regulatory changes and their ability to maintain compliance in a changing regulatory environment.

By conducting thorough due diligence and assessing compliance risks in transactions, organizations can identify potential risks, liabilities, and areas for improvement. This allows them to make informed decisions, negotiate appropriate contractual terms, and develop strategies to mitigate compliance risks effectively. Engaging legal counsel and compliance experts can provide valuable guidance and support throughout the due diligence process.

Integrating Compliance Programs and Cultures Post-merger

Integrating compliance programs and cultures post-merger is crucial to ensure a unified and effective compliance framework in the newly merged entity. Here are key considerations for integrating compliance programs and cultures:

1. **Assess Existing Compliance Programs:** Evaluate the compliance programs of both merging entities to identify strengths, weaknesses, and areas of alignment. Assess the scope, policies, procedures, training, monitoring, and reporting mechanisms of each program. Identify gaps and areas that need to be harmonized to create a unified compliance program.

2. **Define Compliance Objectives and Priorities:** Clearly define the compliance objectives and priorities for the merged entity. This includes identifying the core values, mission, and vision of the compliance program, as well as the key areas of focus based on the compliance risks and regulatory requirements of the industry and jurisdictions of operation.

3. **Establish Integration Teams:** Form cross-functional integration teams comprising representatives from both merging entities. These teams should include compliance professionals, legal experts, HR representatives, and business leaders. Assign responsibilities for integrating compliance programs, aligning policies and procedures, and fostering a unified compliance culture.

4. **Harmonize Policies and Procedures:** Compare the compliance policies and procedures of both entities and identify areas of overlap, inconsistency, or gaps. Develop a harmonization plan to align policies, procedures, and guidelines with a focus on ensuring compliance with relevant laws, regulations, and industry standards. Create a comprehensive set of policies and procedures that reflect the merged entity's values and compliance objectives.

5. **Training and Communication:** Conduct training programs to educate employees on the merged entity's compliance expectations, policies, and procedures. Provide comprehensive training that addresses any changes resulting from the merger, including updates to legal and regulatory requirements. Foster open communication channels to ensure employees

have the necessary information and resources to meet compliance expectations.

6. **Cultural Integration:** Recognize and address cultural differences between the merging entities in terms of compliance practices and expectations. Develop strategies to merge the compliance cultures, taking into account the values and ethics of both entities. Foster a culture of compliance through effective communication, leadership support, and setting the tone at the top.

7. **Consolidate Reporting Mechanisms:** Streamline and consolidate reporting mechanisms to ensure consistent and efficient reporting of compliance concerns. Establish a unified reporting system that encourages employees to report potential violations or compliance issues. Provide clear guidance on reporting channels, confidentiality, and protection against retaliation.

8. **Monitor and Audit Compliance Activities:** Implement monitoring and auditing processes to assess the effectiveness of the integrated compliance program. Conduct regular audits to evaluate compliance with policies, procedures, and regulatory requirements. Monitor compliance metrics, key performance indicators, and incident reporting to identify areas for improvement and address emerging risks.

9. **Provide Ongoing Support and Resources:** Ensure ongoing support and resources for employees to meet compliance expectations. Offer guidance, training, and access to compliance experts who can address specific compliance concerns. Provide channels for employees to seek guidance and clarification on compliance matters.

10. **Continuous Improvement:** Foster a culture of continuous improvement in the integrated compliance program. Encourage feedback from employees and stakeholders to identify areas for enhancement. Regularly review and update the compliance program to adapt to changes in laws, regulations, and industry best practices.

By following these considerations, organizations can effectively integrate compliance programs and cultures post-merger. This integration ensures a unified approach to compliance, mitigates risks, and promotes a strong compliance culture throughout the merged entity. Collaboration, communication, and ongoing monitoring are key to successfully integrating compliance programs and cultures in a post-merger environment.

Compliance Challenges in Consolidating Healthcare Entities

Consolidating healthcare entities presents several compliance challenges that need to be effectively addressed to ensure a smooth transition and continued adherence to applicable laws, regulations, and ethical standards. Here are some common compliance challenges that arise during the consolidation of healthcare entities:

1. **Regulatory Complexity:** Healthcare regulations are complex and vary across jurisdictions and specialties. Consolidating entities may operate in different regions or offer diverse services, requiring a comprehensive understanding of the regulatory landscape. Compliance teams must navigate through the intricacies of multiple regulatory frameworks and ensure compliance with all relevant laws and regulations.

2. **Data Integration and Privacy:** Consolidating healthcare entities often involves merging patient data from various systems. Data integration raises concerns about data privacy and security. Compliance teams must ensure compliance with data protection laws, such as HIPAA, throughout the consolidation process. Robust data sharing agreements and privacy safeguards must be established to protect patient information.

3. **Standardization of Policies and Procedures:** Consolidation brings together different policies, procedures, and practices from each entity. Harmonizing and standardizing these policies and procedures is crucial to ensure consistency and compliance. Compliance teams must assess existing policies and procedures, identify gaps or inconsistencies, and develop unified policies and procedures that reflect regulatory requirements and best practices.

4. **Cultural Alignment:** Consolidating healthcare entities may involve different organizational cultures, approaches to compliance, and ethical standards. Achieving cultural alignment is essential to foster a unified compliance culture and promote ethical conduct. Compliance teams should actively engage with leadership and employees to create a shared vision and values that prioritize compliance and ethical behavior.

5. **Third-Party Relationships:** Consolidation often involves inherited contracts, relationships, and partnerships. Compliance teams must assess the compliance status of these relationships, including vendors, suppliers, and business partners. Due diligence should be conducted to identify potential compliance risks and ensure alignment with the consolidated entity's compliance program and standards.

6. **Workforce Integration:** Consolidation may result in a diverse workforce with varying levels of compliance awareness and training. Ensuring consistent compliance education and training across the consolidated entity is crucial. Compliance teams should develop comprehensive training programs that address the specific compliance requirements, policies, and procedures of the consolidated entity.

7. **Change Management:** Consolidation brings significant changes in processes, systems, and reporting structures. Implementing these changes smoothly requires effective change management strategies. Compliance teams should communicate the purpose and benefits of the consolidation, address employee concerns, and provide support throughout the transition to ensure compliance remains a priority during the change process.

8. **Monitoring and Auditing:** Consolidated entities may face challenges in establishing effective monitoring and auditing processes. Compliance teams must develop robust monitoring and auditing programs that cover all aspects of the consolidated entity's operations. Regular monitoring and audits help identify compliance gaps, address issues promptly, and demonstrate a commitment to compliance and quality.

9. **Integration of IT Systems:** Consolidating entities often involve integrating IT systems, including electronic health record (EHR) systems and other technology platforms. Compliance teams must ensure that IT integration is conducted securely, with appropriate data access controls and safeguards in place. Compliance with data privacy and security regulations, such as HIPAA, must be maintained throughout the integration process.

10. **Ongoing Compliance Management:** Consolidated entities must establish a strong governance structure and ongoing compliance management processes. This includes assigning clear responsibilities, creating reporting mechanisms, conducting regular risk assessments, and implementing compliance monitoring and reporting systems. Compliance should remain a priority even after the consolidation is complete.

Addressing these compliance challenges requires proactive planning, collaboration among stakeholders, and effective communication. Compliance teams must work closely with leadership, legal counsel, and other relevant departments to ensure a smooth consolidation process that upholds regulatory compliance and promotes ethical practices in the consolidated healthcare entity.

Chapter 20

Future Trends and Challenges in Healthcare Compliance

Future trends and challenges in healthcare compliance are shaped by evolving regulations, advancements in technology, and changing industry dynamics. Here are some key trends and challenges that healthcare organizations may face in the coming years:

1. **Evolving Regulatory Landscape:** Healthcare organizations will continue to face the challenge of navigating a complex and ever-changing regulatory landscape. New regulations, amendments to existing laws, and shifts in enforcement priorities will require organizations to stay updated and adapt their compliance programs accordingly. This includes staying abreast of changes in privacy and security regulations, reimbursement policies, and fraud and abuse laws.

2. **Digital Transformation and Health Tech:** The rapid advancement of technology, including telemedicine, artificial intelligence (AI), and wearable devices, introduces new compliance challenges. Healthcare organizations must ensure that their digital systems and technologies comply with privacy and security regulations, data protection laws, and ethical considerations. They must also address issues related to the interoperability of electronic health records (EHRs) and the responsible use of AI and patient-generated health data.

3. **Data Privacy and Cybersecurity:** The increasing volume of patient data, coupled with the rising threat of cyberattacks, makes data privacy and cybersecurity critical compliance concerns. Healthcare organizations must strengthen their data protection measures, implement robust cybersecurity protocols, and comply with privacy regulations such as the General Data Protection Regulation (GDPR) and the Health Insurance Portability and Accountability Act (HIPAA). Safeguarding patient information from unauthorized access and ensuring secure data sharing will remain ongoing challenges.

4. **Increased Focus on Patient-Centric Care:** The shift toward patient-centric care requires healthcare organizations to prioritize patient rights, informed consent, and shared decision-making. Compliance programs must be designed to support patient autonomy, privacy, and dignity. Organizations will need to navigate ethical considerations, legal frameworks, and consent management processes to ensure compliance while delivering patient-centered care.

5. **Value-Based Care and Alternative Payment Models:** The transition from fee-for-service to value-based care models introduces compliance challenges related to reimbursement structures, billing and coding, and quality reporting. Compliance programs must address the requirements of alternative payment models, such as accountable care organizations (ACOs) and bundled payment arrangements, while ensuring accurate documentation, coding, and reporting to support appropriate reimbursement.

6. **Ethics and Social Responsibility:** Healthcare organizations are increasingly expected to uphold ethical standards and demonstrate social responsibility. This includes addressing issues such as equity in healthcare access, diversity and inclusion, and responsible corporate behavior. Compliance programs must encompass ethical guidelines, cultural sensitivity, and socially responsible practices to meet these evolving expectations.

7. **Global Compliance and Cross-Border Operations:** Healthcare organizations expanding their operations internationally face the challenge of complying with diverse regulatory frameworks and cultural norms. Managing compliance in multiple jurisdictions requires a deep understanding of local regulations, data protection laws, and cultural nuances. Organizations must develop global compliance strategies, establish local partnerships, and ensure cross-border compliance while maintaining consistent ethical standards.

8. **Heightened Enforcement and Whistleblower Activity:** Regulatory enforcement efforts and whistleblower activity are expected to increase in the healthcare industry. Government agencies and regulatory bodies will continue to focus on fraud and abuse, data breaches, and compliance violations. Healthcare organizations must be prepared to respond to investigations, implement robust compliance programs, and foster a culture of ethical conduct. Whistleblower protection and effective internal reporting mechanisms will become even more critical.

9. **Supply Chain Integrity:** Ensuring the integrity and compliance of the healthcare supply chain will be a growing challenge. Healthcare organizations must vet and monitor suppliers, manage risks related to counterfeit or substandard products, and comply with regulations governing pharmaceuticals, medical devices, and other supplies. Supply chain transparency and responsible sourcing practices will be increasingly important.

10. **Continuous Monitoring and Auditing:** Traditional compliance monitoring and auditing practices are evolving to embrace data analytics, automation, and continuous monitoring technologies. Healthcare organizations will need to leverage these tools to enhance their compliance monitoring capabilities, identify potential risks in real-time, and proactively address compliance issues. Continuous monitoring and auditing will help organizations stay ahead of compliance challenges and ensure ongoing adherence to regulations.

In summary, future trends and challenges in healthcare compliance revolve around the evolving regulatory landscape, technological advancements, patient-centric care, data privacy and cybersecurity, ethical considerations, global operations, enforcement activities, supply chain integrity, and the need for continuous monitoring and auditing. By staying informed, adopting innovative approaches, and maintaining a proactive compliance mindset, healthcare organizations can navigate these challenges and establish robust compliance programs to safeguard patient safety, privacy, and overall organizational integrity.

Anticipated Regulatory Trends and Changes in the Healthcare Industry

Anticipating regulatory trends and changes in the healthcare industry is crucial for organizations to stay ahead of compliance requirements and adapt their practices accordingly. While specific regulatory trends can vary by region and jurisdiction, here are some anticipated trends and changes in the healthcare industry:

1. **Telehealth and Remote Care:** The COVID-19 pandemic has accelerated the adoption of telehealth and remote care services. Anticipated regulatory trends include the expansion of telehealth reimbursement policies, increased focus on telehealth quality and safety standards, and potential changes in licensure requirements for healthcare professionals practicing across state or international borders.

2. **Data Privacy and Security:** With the increasing digitization of healthcare data and the rising concern over data breaches and privacy violations, regulatory trends will likely focus on strengthening data privacy and security measures. Anticipated changes may include enhanced regulations and enforcement actions related to data protection, patient consent, data breach reporting, and the use of emerging technologies like AI and big data analytics.

3. **Value-Based Care and Alternative Payment Models:** The shift from fee-for-service to value-based care models is expected to continue. Regulatory trends may include the development of new payment models, adjustments to quality reporting requirements, and efforts to streamline the transition to value-based care through regulatory incentives, collaboration, and shared savings programs.

4. **Drug Pricing and Access:** Drug pricing and access have been prominent issues in the healthcare industry. Anticipated regulatory trends may include increased efforts to address rising drug costs, enhance transparency in drug pricing, promote competition, and improve patient access to affordable medications. Additionally, regulatory actions to expedite the approval process for generic and biosimilar drugs may be anticipated.

5. **Artificial Intelligence (AI) and Digital Health:** The integration of AI and digital health technologies into healthcare delivery and decision-making processes is expected to continue. Anticipated regulatory trends may include the development of guidelines or regulations to ensure the safe and ethical use of AI in healthcare, address potential biases in AI algorithms, and establish standards for the evaluation and validation of digital health solutions.

6. **Cybersecurity and Data Protection:** As the healthcare industry becomes increasingly digitized, the risk of cyber threats and data breaches rises. Anticipated regulatory trends may include stricter cybersecurity regulations, requirements for risk assessments and incident response planning, and increased focus on third-party vendor management to ensure data protection throughout the healthcare ecosystem.

7. **Interoperability and Health Information Exchange:** The seamless exchange of health information among healthcare systems and providers is a priority for improving care coordination and patient outcomes. Anticipated regulatory trends may focus on promoting interoperability standards, enforcing data sharing requirements, and facilitating secure health information exchange between organizations and across different health IT systems.

8. **Compliance Enforcement and Anti-Fraud Measures:** Regulatory authorities are expected to maintain a strong focus on compliance enforcement and anti-fraud measures. Anticipated trends may include increased investigations, audits, and penalties for non-compliance, as well as efforts to strengthen whistleblower protections and incentives for reporting fraud and abuse.

9. **Social Determinants of Health:** There is growing recognition of the impact of social determinants of health on patient outcomes. Anticipated regulatory trends may include efforts to address social determinants of health through regulatory initiatives, funding programs, and collaborations with community-based organizations to promote health equity and improve population health outcomes.

10. **International Collaboration and Harmonization:** Given the global nature of healthcare and the increasing interconnectedness of healthcare systems, anticipated regulatory trends may involve greater international collaboration and harmonization of regulations. Efforts may include aligning standards, sharing best practices, and facilitating mutual recognition of regulatory approvals to streamline international operations and enhance patient safety.

It's important for healthcare organizations to closely monitor regulatory developments, engage with industry associations and regulatory bodies, and proactively adapt their compliance programs to meet evolving requirements. By staying informed and anticipating these regulatory trends and changes, organizations can position themselves to navigate compliance challenges effectively and ensure they remain compliant with the evolving regulatory landscape in the healthcare industry.

Impact of Technology Advancements on Compliance (AI, Blockchain, Telehealth)

Technology advancements, such as artificial intelligence (AI), blockchain, and telehealth, have a significant impact on compliance in the healthcare industry. Here's an overview of their implications:

1. **Artificial Intelligence (AI):** AI technologies have the potential to revolutionize compliance by automating processes, analyzing large datasets, and identifying patterns that may indicate compliance risks or anomalies. AI-powered tools can assist in monitoring and detecting fraud, waste, and abuse in billing and coding practices, improving accuracy and efficiency in compliance auditing

and monitoring. However, the use of AI also brings challenges related to transparency, algorithmic bias, and data privacy, requiring organizations to carefully consider ethical and regulatory implications.

2. **Blockchain Technology:** Blockchain technology offers enhanced data security, transparency, and traceability, which can significantly impact compliance in healthcare. Blockchain can facilitate secure sharing of healthcare data, streamline identity verification, and provide a tamper-resistant record of transactions. It can help address compliance challenges related to data privacy, consent management, and data integrity. Blockchain-enabled smart contracts can automate compliance processes and enforce contractual obligations, reducing the need for intermediaries and enhancing compliance efficiency.

3. **Telehealth and Remote Care:** The rapid expansion of telehealth and remote care services introduces compliance considerations related to privacy, security, and regulatory compliance. Telehealth platforms must adhere to data privacy regulations, such as HIPAA, to ensure the confidentiality and security of patient information. Compliance programs should address the unique risks associated with telehealth, such as proper patient authentication, appropriate licensure and credentialing of healthcare professionals across state or international borders, and ensuring the quality and safety of telehealth services.

Technology advancements have the potential to enhance compliance efforts by streamlining processes, improving data security, and enabling more efficient monitoring and auditing. However, healthcare organizations must also address associated challenges, such as ensuring the ethical use of AI, managing data privacy and consent issues, and adapting compliance programs to account for the unique risks introduced by these technologies. It is essential to strike a balance between leveraging technology's benefits while mitigating any potential risks to maintain compliance and uphold patient trust in the healthcare system.

Addressing Emerging Compliance Challenges and Risks

Addressing emerging compliance challenges and risks requires proactive measures and a strategic approach. Here are some key steps to address these challenges:

1. **Stay Informed and Updated:** Regularly monitor regulatory developments, industry trends, and emerging risks to stay informed about new compliance

challenges. Engage with industry associations, regulatory bodies, and professional networks to stay updated on best practices, guidelines, and changes in regulations.

2. **Conduct Risk Assessments:** Perform comprehensive risk assessments to identify emerging compliance risks specific to your organization. Assess internal processes, external factors, and industry trends that may impact compliance. Prioritize risks based on their potential impact and likelihood, and develop strategies to mitigate them effectively.

3. **Enhance Compliance Training and Education:** Provide ongoing training and education programs to employees at all levels to increase awareness of emerging compliance challenges and risks. Offer targeted training on specific topics, such as data privacy, cybersecurity, telehealth compliance, or new regulatory requirements. Ensure that employees have the knowledge and tools to adhere to compliance standards.

4. **Strengthen Data Privacy and Security:** As technology evolves, the importance of data privacy and security increases. Implement robust data protection measures, including encryption, access controls, and regular security assessments. Stay updated on data privacy regulations and ensure compliance with requirements such as HIPAA, GDPR, or other applicable laws.

5. **Foster a Compliance Culture:** Promote a culture of compliance throughout the organization by fostering ethical behavior, accountability, and transparency. Establish clear expectations for compliance and provide channels for employees to report concerns or seek guidance. Encourage open communication, provide regular compliance updates, and recognize and reward ethical conduct.

6. **Adapt Compliance Programs:** Continuously assess and adapt compliance programs to address emerging risks. Regularly review and update policies, procedures, and controls to align with new regulatory requirements and emerging industry trends. Incorporate new compliance frameworks and best practices to address specific challenges, such as telehealth compliance or AI governance.

7. **Leverage Technology Solutions:** Explore technology solutions, such as compliance management software, data analytics tools, and automated monitoring systems, to streamline compliance processes and enhance risk management. Use technology to monitor and detect potential compliance breaches, automate compliance reporting, and facilitate data analysis for proactive risk mitigation.

8. **Foster Collaboration and Partnerships:** Engage with industry peers, compliance professionals, and external experts to share knowledge, best practices, and insights into emerging compliance challenges. Collaborate with legal counsel, consultants, and regulatory bodies to navigate complex compliance issues and obtain guidance on addressing emerging risks.

9. **Monitor and Evaluate Compliance Performance:** Implement regular monitoring and auditing processes to assess compliance performance and identify areas for improvement. Conduct internal audits, risk assessments, and compliance reviews to detect potential gaps or weaknesses. Use the findings to implement corrective actions, strengthen controls, and enhance compliance effectiveness.

10. **Establish Effective Reporting and Investigation Mechanisms:** Implement robust reporting and investigation mechanisms to encourage employees to report potential compliance violations or emerging risks. Ensure confidentiality, non-retaliation, and protection for whistleblowers. Promptly investigate reported concerns and take appropriate actions to address any identified compliance issues.

By taking a proactive and comprehensive approach to addressing emerging compliance challenges and risks, healthcare organizations can strengthen their compliance programs, mitigate potential risks, and maintain regulatory compliance in a rapidly evolving healthcare landscape.

Strategies for Future-proofing Compliance Programs

Future-proofing compliance programs involves implementing strategies that anticipate and adapt to changes in the regulatory, technological, and operational landscape. Here are some strategies to consider:

1. **Stay Agile and Adaptive:** Build flexibility into your compliance program to quickly respond to evolving regulations and industry trends. Regularly assess and update compliance policies, procedures, and controls to address new requirements and emerging risks.

2. **Embrace Technology Solutions:** Leverage technology to enhance compliance effectiveness. Implement compliance management systems, data analytics tools, and automated monitoring systems to streamline compliance processes, identify potential risks, and facilitate real-time reporting and analysis.

3. **Foster a Compliance Culture:** Cultivate a strong culture of compliance across the organization. Ensure that ethical behavior, accountability, and compliance awareness are ingrained in the organization's values and reflected in employee behavior. Encourage open communication and provide training and resources to foster a compliance mindset at all levels.

4. **Conduct Regular Risk Assessments:** Perform comprehensive risk assessments to identify emerging compliance risks. Evaluate internal processes, external factors, and industry trends that may impact compliance. Prioritize risks and develop strategies to mitigate them effectively.

5. **Enhance Training and Education:** Provide ongoing training and education programs to ensure employees are equipped with the knowledge and skills necessary to navigate evolving compliance challenges. Offer specialized training on emerging compliance topics, such as data privacy, cybersecurity, and emerging regulations.

6. **Engage in Regulatory Monitoring and Advocacy:** Stay abreast of regulatory developments and engage with industry associations and regulatory bodies. Participate in relevant forums and advocacy efforts to influence the development of regulations and standards that align with your organization's needs and compliance goals.

7. **Foster Collaboration and Partnerships:** Collaborate with other industry stakeholders, compliance professionals, and external experts to share knowledge, best practices, and insights. Build partnerships with legal counsel, consultants, and regulatory bodies to navigate complex compliance issues and obtain guidance on emerging risks.

8. **Implement Continuous Monitoring and Auditing:** Utilize technology and data analytics to implement continuous monitoring and auditing processes. Regularly monitor compliance metrics, conduct internal audits, and perform proactive risk assessments to detect potential compliance gaps and address them promptly.

9. **Establish Effective Reporting and Investigation Mechanisms:** Implement robust reporting and investigation mechanisms to encourage employees to report potential compliance violations or emerging risks. Ensure confidentiality, non-retaliation, and protection for whistleblowers. Promptly investigate reported concerns and take appropriate actions to address any identified compliance issues.

10. **Maintain Strong Governance and Oversight:** Ensure the compliance program has strong governance and oversight mechanisms. Assign clear responsibilities, establish reporting lines, and regularly review the effectiveness of the compliance program. Senior leadership should actively demonstrate commitment to compliance and provide necessary resources for its implementation.

By implementing these strategies, healthcare organizations can future-proof their compliance programs, enabling them to effectively adapt to regulatory changes, technological advancements, and emerging risks. This proactive approach helps organizations maintain regulatory compliance, mitigate risks, and foster a culture of integrity and ethics.

Conclusion

n conclusion, regulatory compliance in the healthcare industry is a complex and ever-evolving landscape that poses numerous challenges for organizations. Compliance with healthcare regulations is of utmost importance as it ensures patient safety, protects sensitive information, promotes ethical practices, and mitigates legal and financial risks. Key regulatory bodies, such as the FDA, CMS, HIPAA, and others, play crucial roles in enforcing compliance and setting standards.

Healthcare organizations face various complexities, including regulatory requirements, data privacy and security, quality and patient safety, billing and coding compliance, pharmaceutical and medical device regulations, research and clinical trials compliance, and more. Building a robust compliance program is essential, which involves establishing policies and procedures, conducting risk assessments, implementing internal controls, and training employees.

Compliance officers play a vital role in overseeing compliance efforts, ensuring adherence to regulations, conducting audits, and managing investigations. They are responsible for monitoring regulatory changes, developing compliance strategies, and fostering a culture of compliance within the organization.

The healthcare industry is continuously evolving, and emerging trends and developments impact compliance practices. These include advancements in technology such as AI, telemedicine, and wearables, as well as international regulations and global compliance challenges.

Building a compliance program requires attention to detail, adaptability, and a commitment to ongoing improvement. It involves addressing various components such as privacy and security, quality improvement, billing and coding, pharmaceutical and medical device regulations, research and clinical trials, health information technology, health insurance and payer relations, long-term care facilities, fraud investigations, and more.

By proactively addressing compliance challenges, staying updated with regulations, leveraging technology, fostering a culture of compliance, and collaborating with industry stakeholders, healthcare organizations can navigate the complexities of regulatory compliance successfully. Future-proofing compliance programs involves anticipating regulatory trends, addressing emerging risks, and implementing strategies to adapt to evolving regulatory and technological landscapes.

Overall, compliance in the healthcare industry is a critical function that ensures ethical conduct, patient safety, and legal compliance. By prioritizing compliance and implementing robust compliance programs, healthcare organizations can operate with integrity, mitigate risks, and provide high-quality care in a complex and highly regulated environment.

Recap of Key Concepts Covered in the Book

Throughout the book, we have explored various key concepts related to regulatory compliance in the healthcare industry. Here is a recap of the key concepts covered:

1. Regulatory Compliance: Regulatory compliance refers to the adherence of healthcare organizations to laws, regulations, and standards set by regulatory bodies such as the FDA, CMS, HIPAA, and others. Compliance ensures patient safety, protects sensitive information, and mitigates legal and financial risks.

2. Key Regulatory Bodies: We discussed the roles and responsibilities of key regulatory bodies, including the FDA (Food and Drug Administration), CMS (Centers for Medicare and Medicaid Services), HIPAA (Health Insurance Portability and Accountability Act), and others. These regulatory bodies enforce compliance and set standards in areas such as drug approval, healthcare billing and coding, data privacy, and more.

3. Compliance Challenges: Healthcare organizations face various complexities and challenges, including navigating a complex regulatory landscape, ensuring data privacy and security, maintaining quality and patient safety standards, addressing billing and coding compliance, complying with pharmaceutical and medical device regulations, and managing compliance in research and clinical trials.

4. Building a Compliance Program: We discussed the essential components of a robust compliance program, including establishing policies, procedures, and internal controls, conducting risk assessments, implementing auditing

and monitoring processes, and training employees on compliance requirements.

5. Role of Compliance Officers: Compliance officers play a crucial role in overseeing compliance efforts, managing compliance programs, monitoring regulatory changes, conducting audits, and ensuring adherence to regulations. They are responsible for developing compliance strategies, fostering a culture of compliance, and managing investigations.

6. Healthcare Privacy and Security Regulations: We explored healthcare privacy laws, such as HIPAA and the HITECH Act, which regulate the protection of patient health information and ensure data security. We discussed the importance of ensuring patient confidentiality, implementing safeguards for electronic health records (EHR), and responding to data breaches.

7. Quality and Patient Safety Standards: We examined quality improvement initiatives in healthcare, including compliance with quality standards, patient safety regulations, strategies for error prevention, monitoring adverse events, and implementing root cause analysis to enhance patient safety and care outcomes.

8. Billing and Coding Compliance: We covered billing and coding regulations, such as CMS guidelines, CPT codes, and ICD-10, which ensure accurate billing and reimbursement processes. We discussed the importance of accurate coding and documentation practices, strategies for preventing fraud and abuse, and conducting internal and external audits.

9. Pharmaceutical and Medical Device Regulations: We explored regulatory requirements for pharmaceuticals and medical devices, including FDA regulations for drug approval processes, post-marketing surveillance, medical device classification, pre-market clearance, product safety, labeling, and advertising compliance.

10. Compliance in Research and Clinical Trials: We discussed compliance challenges in research and clinical trials, including ethical considerations, compliance with human subjects protection regulations, informed consent, privacy concerns, monitoring and auditing clinical trials, and addressing research misconduct.

11. Compliance in a Changing Healthcare Landscape: We examined the impact of healthcare reforms and policy changes on regulatory compliance,

emerging technologies such as telemedicine, AI, and wearables, international regulations and global compliance challenges, and strategies for staying updated with regulatory changes.

12. Training and Education for Compliance: We emphasized the importance of training and education in promoting compliance, designing effective compliance training programs, engaging employees in compliance initiatives, and continuous professional development for compliance professionals.

13. Case Studies and Best Practices: We discussed real-world case studies highlighting compliance challenges and their resolutions, best practices for achieving and maintaining regulatory compliance, and lessons learned from successful compliance programs.

14. Compliance in Health Information Technology: We explored compliance considerations in health information technology, including regulatory requirements for HIT systems, EHR interoperability, health information privacy, and security, and compliance challenges in implementing and maintaining HIT systems.

15. Compliance in Health Insurance and Payer Relations: We examined health insurance regulations such as the Affordable Care Act (ACA) and ERISA, compliance requirements for insurance companies and payers, ensuring accurate claims processing and reimbursement, and addressing compliance challenges in payer-provider relationships.

16. Compliance in Long-Term Care Facilities: We discussed regulatory considerations specific to long-term care facilities, compliance with nursing home regulations including CMS guidelines and OIG recommendations, ensuring quality of care and resident rights, and addressing compliance challenges in long-term care settings.

17. Compliance and Healthcare Fraud Investigations: We explored the overview of healthcare fraud and abuse investigations, the role of government agencies such as the DOJ and OIG in enforcing compliance, whistleblower protections, the False Claims Act, and responding to investigations and managing legal implications.

18. Compliance Auditing and Monitoring: We highlighted the importance of regular auditing and monitoring in compliance programs, developing an effective auditing and monitoring framework, conducting internal

audits, implementing corrective actions, and leveraging data analytics for compliance monitoring and risk assessment.

19. Compliance in Medical Ethics and Research Misconduct: We discussed ethical considerations in medical practice and research, compliance with ethical guidelines and principles such as the Nuremberg Code and Belmont Report, addressing research misconduct and ethical violations, and the role of Institutional Review Boards (IRBs) in promoting compliance.

20. Compliance and Corporate Governance: We explored the integration of compliance into corporate governance structures, compliance considerations for the board of directors and executive management, transparency and accountability in compliance reporting, and the role of compliance in promoting organizational integrity and ethics.

21. Compliance in Global Healthcare Operations: We discussed international regulations and standards for healthcare compliance, navigating cultural and legal differences in global compliance, strategies for managing compliance across international operations, and addressing corruption risks and implementing anti-bribery measures.

Throughout the book, we have covered a wide range of topics to provide a comprehensive understanding of regulatory compliance in the healthcare industry. By considering these key concepts, healthcare organizations can navigate the complexities of compliance, mitigate risks, and ensure adherence to regulatory requirements to promote patient safety, protect sensitive information, and maintain the integrity of their operations.

Final Thoughts on the Importance of Regulatory Compliance in Healthcare

In conclusion, regulatory compliance is of utmost importance in the healthcare industry. Compliance ensures patient safety, protects sensitive information, promotes ethical practices, and mitigates legal and financial risks for healthcare organizations. The complex and ever-evolving regulatory landscape poses numerous challenges, requiring organizations to stay updated, proactive, and adaptable.

Compliance is not just a legal obligation but also a moral and ethical responsibility. It establishes trust with patients, regulators, and the public by demonstrating a commitment to delivering high-quality care and upholding ethical standards.

Non-compliance can have severe consequences, including financial penalties, reputational damage, loss of patient trust, and even criminal charges.

Healthcare organizations must establish robust compliance programs that encompass policies, procedures, internal controls, training, auditing, and monitoring. Compliance officers play a crucial role in overseeing these programs, ensuring adherence to regulations, and managing investigations. A strong compliance culture should permeate throughout the organization, with accountability and transparency at its core.

The healthcare industry is constantly evolving, with emerging technologies, changing regulations, and shifting healthcare delivery models. This necessitates a proactive approach to compliance, anticipating and addressing emerging risks, and staying abreast of regulatory changes. It also requires organizations to leverage technology, foster collaboration, and continuously improve their compliance programs.

By prioritizing regulatory compliance, healthcare organizations can safeguard patient safety, protect sensitive information, and maintain the trust and confidence of patients, regulators, and stakeholders. Compliance is an integral part of delivering quality care, ensuring ethical practices, and contributing to the overall integrity and sustainability of the healthcare industry.

Encouragement for Ongoing Commitment to Compliance

As we conclude our discussion on regulatory compliance in the healthcare industry, we would like to emphasize the importance of ongoing commitment to compliance. Compliance is not a one-time effort but an ongoing journey that requires continuous dedication and vigilance.

We encourage healthcare organizations to prioritize compliance as a fundamental aspect of their operations. Embed compliance into the fabric of your organization by fostering a culture of integrity, ethics, and accountability. Engage employees at all levels, from frontline staff to senior leadership, in the importance of compliance and their roles in upholding it.

Stay informed about regulatory changes, emerging risks, and best practices in compliance. Regularly assess your compliance program, conduct audits, and identify areas for improvement. Leverage technology solutions and data analytics to enhance compliance monitoring, risk assessment, and reporting capabilities.

Invest in training and education to ensure that employees are equipped with the knowledge and skills necessary to navigate compliance challenges. Provide resources, guidance, and support to employees to encourage reporting of potential compliance issues and address them promptly.

Collaborate with industry peers, regulatory bodies, and compliance professionals to share insights, learn from best practices, and stay ahead of emerging compliance trends. Participate in industry forums, conferences, and working groups to stay connected with the latest developments.

Remember that compliance is not just about meeting regulatory requirements; it is about doing what is right for patients, employees, and the community. By maintaining a strong commitment to compliance, you demonstrate your dedication to providing safe, high-quality care and upholding ethical standards.

We commend your ongoing commitment to compliance in the healthcare industry. Together, we can ensure the integrity, trust, and sustainability of the healthcare system, ultimately benefiting patients and society as a whole.

Resources for Further Information and Assistance

For further information and assistance on regulatory compliance in the healthcare industry, here are some resources that you may find helpful:

1. Regulatory Bodies: Visit the websites of regulatory bodies such as the FDA (Food and Drug Administration), CMS (Centers for Medicare and Medicaid Services), HHS (U.S. Department of Health and Human Services), OCR (Office for Civil Rights), and OIG (Office of Inspector General) for official guidelines, regulations, and resources.

2. Industry Associations: Join industry associations and organizations that focus on healthcare compliance, such as the Healthcare Compliance Association (HCCA), the American Health Lawyers Association (AHLA), or the American Medical Association (AMA). These associations provide access to valuable resources, educational materials, networking opportunities, and conferences.

3. Professional Networks: Engage with professional networks and forums to connect with other compliance professionals and exchange insights. Platforms like LinkedIn and professional online communities dedicated to

healthcare compliance can provide valuable information, discussions, and resources.

4. Training and Certification Programs: Explore training and certification programs in healthcare compliance offered by reputable organizations. These programs can enhance your knowledge and skills in specific compliance areas and provide a recognized credential. Examples include the Certified in Healthcare Compliance (CHC) certification by the HCCA and the Certified Professional in Healthcare Compliance (CPHCTM) certification by the Compliance Certification Board (CCB).

5. Publications and Journals: Stay updated with the latest trends and developments in healthcare compliance by reading industry publications and journals. Some notable publications include Compliance Today, Journal of Healthcare Compliance, and Health Affairs.

6. Webinars and Podcasts: Attend webinars or listen to podcasts focused on healthcare compliance. These platforms often feature experts who share insights, best practices, and practical tips on compliance-related topics.

7. Legal Counsel and Consultants: Seek guidance from legal counsel specializing in healthcare law or consultants with expertise in healthcare compliance. They can provide tailored advice, assist with compliance program development, and support your organization in navigating complex compliance challenges.

8. Government Websites: Government websites such as the Federal Register, the Department of Health and Human Services (HHS) website, and the Office for Civil Rights (OCR) website offer resources, guidance, and updates on regulatory requirements and compliance initiatives.

9. Healthcare Compliance Websites: Many organizations and firms have dedicated websites that offer resources, articles, and guidance on healthcare compliance. Examples include the Health Care Compliance Association (HCCA), the Society of Corporate Compliance and Ethics (SCCE), and the American Health Information Management Association (AHIMA).

10. Government Compliance Programs: Government agencies, such as the Department of Justice (DOJ) and the Office of Inspector General (OIG), have established compliance program guidance for various sectors of the healthcare industry. These resources can provide valuable insights into building effective compliance programs. For example, the DOJ's "Evaluation

of Corporate Compliance Programs" and the OIG's "Compliance Program Guidance for Hospitals" are valuable resources.

11. Compliance Networks and Forums: Joining compliance networks and forums can provide opportunities for networking, knowledge sharing, and collaboration with other compliance professionals. Platforms like ComplianceOnline, ComplianceNet, and LinkedIn groups dedicated to healthcare compliance can connect you with a community of professionals in the field.

12. Healthcare Compliance Conferences and Events: Attend healthcare compliance conferences and events to stay updated on the latest trends, best practices, and regulatory changes. These events often feature industry experts and provide opportunities for learning and networking. Some notable conferences include the HCCA Compliance Institute and the SCCE Compliance and Ethics Institute.

13. Government Advisory and Guidance Materials: Government agencies regularly publish advisory opinions, guidance documents, and enforcement actions related to healthcare compliance. These resources can provide insights into compliance expectations and help organizations align their practices accordingly. Check the websites of regulatory bodies such as the FDA, CMS, and OCR for such materials.

14. Healthcare Compliance Software and Tools: Explore compliance software and tools designed specifically for the healthcare industry. These solutions can help streamline compliance processes, manage documentation, automate monitoring, and enhance reporting capabilities. Examples include compliance management software, data privacy tools, and auditing tools.

15. Compliance Research and Whitepapers: Conduct research and access industry-specific whitepapers and research studies that delve into healthcare compliance. These resources often provide in-depth analysis, best practices, and insights into emerging trends. Academic journals, think tanks, and research organizations in the healthcare field are good sources for such materials.

Appendix

Glossary of Key Terms and Acronyms

TERMS	DEFINITIONS
Anti-Kickback Statute	A federal law that prohibits the exchange of remuneration to induce or reward referrals for services reimbursed by federal healthcare programs
Anti-Kickback Statute	A federal law that prohibits the exchange of remuneration in return for referrals for services reimbursed by federal healthcare programs, such as Medicare and Medicaid
Auditing	Systematic examination and evaluation of organizational processes, activities, and records to ensure compliance, identify weaknesses, and detect any non-compliant practices
Business Associate Agreement (BAA)	A contract required by HIPAA that outlines the responsibilities and obligations of a business associate who handles protected health information on behalf of a covered entity
CHC (Certified in Healthcare Compliance)	A professional certification offered by the Health Care Compliance Association (HCCA) for individuals who demonstrate expertise in healthcare compliance
CLIA (Clinical Laboratory Improvement Amendments)	Federal standards that regulate clinical laboratories and ensure the accuracy and reliability of laboratory testing
CMS (Centers for Medicare and Medicaid Services)	A federal agency within the U.S. Department of Health and Human Services that administers Medicare and Medicaid programs and establishes regulations and guidelines related to healthcare reimbursement

TERMS	DEFINITIONS
Code of Conduct	A set of principles, values, and ethical standards that guide the behavior and decision-making of individuals within an organization
Compliance	The adherence to laws, regulations, and standards to ensure ethical and legal practices within the healthcare industry
Compliance Culture	The values, attitudes, and behaviors within an organization that prioritize and promote ethical conduct, compliance with laws and regulations, and a commitment to integrity
Compliance Dashboard	A visual representation or summary of key compliance metrics, activities, and performance indicators to provide a snapshot of an organization's compliance status
Compliance Gap Analysis	An assessment conducted to identify gaps or deficiencies in an organization's compliance program compared to regulatory requirements and best practices
Compliance Gap Remediation	Actions taken to address identified gaps or deficiencies in an organization's compliance program, controls, or processes
Compliance Hotline	A confidential reporting mechanism established by organizations to allow employees and other stakeholders to report compliance concerns, potential violations, or unethical behavior
Compliance Monitoring	Ongoing oversight and review of organizational activities, processes, and controls to assess compliance with laws, regulations, and internal policies
Compliance Officer	An individual responsible for overseeing and managing compliance efforts within an organization, including developing policies, conducting audits, and ensuring adherence to regulations

TERMS	DEFINITIONS
Compliance Reporting	The process of documenting and reporting compliance-related incidents, concerns, or violations to appropriate channels, such as the compliance officer, management, or through a compliance hotline
Compliance Risk	The likelihood and potential impact of noncompliance with laws, regulations, or organizational policies, which can result in negative consequences for the organization
Conflict of Interest	A situation in which an individual's personal or financial interests conflict with their professional duties or responsibilities, potentially compromising impartiality or objectivity
Corporate Compliance Program	A comprehensive framework implemented by organizations to promote adherence to laws, regulations, and ethical standards. It includes policies, procedures, and processes to prevent, detect, and respond to noncompliance.
Corporate Integrity Agreement (CIA)	A contractual agreement between a healthcare organization and the government, typically as part of a settlement, in which the organization agrees to specific compliance obligations and oversight
Data Breach	Unauthorized access, use, or disclosure of protected health information, which compromises the privacy and security of individuals' health data
Data Encryption	The process of converting sensitive information into a code to prevent unauthorized access or disclosure
DEA (Drug Enforcement Administration)	A federal agency responsible for enforcing controlled substances laws and regulations in the United States
Due Diligence	The process of thoroughly researching and assessing the compliance history, reputation, and financial stability of an organization or individual before entering into a business relationship or transaction

TERMS	DEFINITIONS
EHR (Electronic Health Records)	Digital versions of patients' medical records that are stored and accessed electronically, facilitating the management and exchange of health information
External Audit	An independent evaluation of an organization's financial statements, controls, and compliance with regulations by a certified public accounting firm or regulatory authority
False Claims Act	A federal law that imposes liability on individuals or entities that submit false or fraudulent claims for payment to the government
FDA (Food and Drug Administration)	A regulatory agency in the United States responsible for ensuring the safety and efficacy of food, drugs, and medical devices
Fraud, Waste, and Abuse (FWA)	Activities that involve intentional deception or misuse of resources within the healthcare system, resulting in financial losses or harm to individuals
Fraudulent Billing	Intentional submission of false or misleading information in claims or billing processes to obtain improper reimbursement from healthcare payers
GMP (Good Manufacturing Practice)	Guidelines and standards that ensure the quality and consistency of pharmaceutical products during manufacturing, packaging, and distribution
HCCA (Health Care Compliance Association)	A professional association that provides resources, education, and networking opportunities for healthcare compliance professionals
HEDIS (Healthcare Effectiveness Data and Information Set)	A set of performance measures used by health plans to assess the quality of care and services provided to their members
HIPAA (Health Insurance Portability and Accountability Act)	A federal law in the United States that protects the privacy and security of individuals' health information and establishes standards for electronic health transactions

TERMS	DEFINITIONS
HITECH Act (Health Information Technology for Economic and Clinical Health Act)	A federal law in the United States that promotes the adoption and meaningful use of electronic health records (EHR) and strengthens privacy and security protections for health information
ICD-10 (International Classification of Diseases, Tenth Revision)	A coding system used to classify and code diagnoses, symptoms, and procedures for medical billing and reporting purposes
Incident Response Plan	A predetermined plan of action that outlines steps to be taken in the event of a compliance incident or breach, including containment, investigation, communication, and resolution
Independent Review Organization (IRO)	An external entity hired to assess an organization's compliance with regulations, contractual obligations, or settlement agreements
Internal Controls	Processes, policies, and procedures implemented by an organization to ensure compliance, protect assets, and minimize the risk of fraud or errors
IRB (Institutional Review Board)	An independent committee that reviews and approves research studies involving human subjects to ensure compliance with ethical guidelines and protect participants' rights and welfare
NIST (National Institute of Standards and Technology)	A federal agency that develops and promotes standards, including cybersecurity frameworks, to enhance the security and privacy of sensitive information
Noncompliance	Failure to adhere to applicable laws, regulations, or organizational policies, leading to potential legal, financial, or reputational risks
NPI (National Provider Identifier)	A unique identification number assigned to healthcare providers in the United States for standardized identification and billing purposes
OCR (Office for Civil Rights)	A division of the U.S. Department of Health and Human Services that enforces the privacy and security regulations under HIPAA

TERMS	DEFINITIONS
OIG (Office of Inspector General)	An independent office within the U.S. Department of Health and Human Services responsible for preventing fraud, waste, and abuse in federal healthcare programs
OSHA (Occupational Safety and Health Administration)	A federal agency that sets and enforces workplace safety and health regulations to ensure safe working conditions for employees
PHI (Personal Health Information)	Similar to PHI, it refers to individually identifiable health information that is protected under various privacy laws
PHI (Protected Health Information)	Individually identifiable health information that is protected under HIPAA and includes demographic, medical, and financial information
Privacy Rule	The HIPAA Privacy Rule sets standards for the use and disclosure of individuals' protected health information and grants individuals certain rights over their health information
Regulatory Body	An organization or government agency responsible for creating and enforcing regulations and standards in the healthcare industry
Remediation	The process of correcting or addressing compliance deficiencies or violations identified through audits, investigations, or monitoring activities
Risk Assessment	The process of identifying, analyzing, and evaluating potential risks and vulnerabilities within an organization to determine their potential impact and likelihood
Risk Management	The identification, assessment, and mitigation of risks to minimize the likelihood of compliance failures, financial losses, reputational damage, and other negative consequences
Sanctions	Penalties or punitive actions imposed on individuals or organizations for noncompliance with laws, regulations, or contractual obligations

TERMS	DEFINITIONS
Security Rule	The HIPAA Security Rule establishes safeguards to protect electronic protected health information and sets requirements for ensuring its confidentiality, integrity, and availability
Stark Law (Physician Self-Referral Law)	A federal law that prohibits physicians from referring Medicare or Medicaid patients to entities with which they have a financial relationship, unless specific exceptions are met
Stark Law (Physician Self-Referral Law)	A federal law that prohibits physicians from referring Medicare or Medicaid patients for designated health services to entities with which they have a financial relationship, unless an exception applies
Third-Party Risk Management	The process of assessing and managing the compliance risks associated with engaging and relying on third-party vendors, suppliers, or business partners
Whistleblower	An individual who reports illegal or unethical activities within an organization to authorities or other appropriate entities

Sample Compliance Program Templates

Here are some elements commonly found in compliance program templates and checklists:

1. Program Structure and Oversight:

    - Designation of a compliance officer or compliance team responsible for program implementation and oversight.

    - Establishment of a compliance committee or advisory group to provide guidance and support.

2. Written Policies and Procedures:

    - Development of comprehensive policies and procedures that address regulatory requirements and organizational standards.

- Documentation of processes for risk assessment, training and education, incident reporting, and monitoring.

3. Code of Conduct and Ethics:

   - Creation of a code of conduct that outlines the organization's commitment to compliance and ethical behavior.

   - Communication and distribution of the code of conduct to all employees and stakeholders.

4. Training and Education:

   - Implementation of regular training programs to educate employees on compliance policies, procedures, and regulations.

   - Documentation of training sessions and tracking of employee completion and understanding.

5. Risk Assessment and Management:

   - Conducting periodic risk assessments to identify potential compliance risks and vulnerabilities.

   - Development of risk mitigation strategies and action plans to address identified risks.

6. Monitoring and Auditing:

   - Establishment of a monitoring and auditing program to assess compliance with policies and regulations.

   - Conducting regular internal audits and assessments to identify areas of noncompliance and implement corrective actions.

7. Reporting and Incident Management:

   - Implementation of a confidential reporting mechanism, such as a compliance hotline, for employees to report compliance concerns or violations.

   - Development of processes for the timely investigation and resolution of reported incidents.

8. Enforcement and Disciplinary Actions:

   - Establishing disciplinary policies and procedures to address noncompliance.

   - Ensuring consistent enforcement of compliance standards and appropriate consequences for violations.

9. Vendor and Third-Party Due Diligence:

- Implementing processes to assess and monitor compliance of vendors and third-party entities.

- Conducting due diligence on potential vendors to ensure they align with compliance requirements.

10. Documentation and Recordkeeping:

- Maintaining accurate and complete documentation of compliance activities, including policies, training records, audits, and incident reports.

  Establishing processes for record retention and accessibility.

11. Continuous Improvement:

- Committing to ongoing evaluation and enhancement of the compliance program based on changing regulations, industry best practices, and identified areas for improvement.

- Periodic review and update of policies, procedures, and training materials to ensure their relevance and effectiveness.

Relevant Regulatory Guidelines and Resources

Here are some relevant regulatory guidelines and resources that can provide guidance and information on healthcare compliance:

1. U.S. Department of Health and Human Services (HHS):

- Office of Inspector General (OIG): The OIG provides guidance, reports, and resources related to healthcare fraud, waste, and abuse prevention, as well as compliance program guidance.

- Office for Civil Rights (OCR): The OCR offers guidance on HIPAA privacy and security regulations, including resources on breach notification, patient rights, and safeguards for protected health information (PHI).

2. Centers for Medicare and Medicaid Services (CMS):

- CMS Compliance Program Guidance: CMS provides guidance and resources on compliance program requirements for various healthcare settings, including hospitals, nursing homes, and home health agencies.

- Medicare Learning Network (MLN): MLN offers educational resources, guidelines, and updates on Medicare billing and coding compliance.

3. Food and Drug Administration (FDA):

- FDA Regulatory Guidance: The FDA provides guidance documents, regulations, and resources related to drug approvals, medical device regulations, manufacturing practices, and clinical trials.

4. Office of the National Coordinator for Health Information Technology (ONC):

- ONC Health IT Certification Program: ONC offers resources and guidance related to health IT, interoperability, and the certification of electronic health record (EHR) systems.

5. Office for Human Research Protections (OHRP):

- OHRP Guidance: OHRP provides guidance and resources on the ethical conduct of research involving human subjects, including regulations and compliance requirements.

6. National Institutes of Health (NIH):

- NIH Office of Extramural Research (OER): The OER offers resources and guidelines on the responsible conduct of research, grant management, and compliance with NIH policies and regulations.

7. International Organization for Standardization (ISO):

- ISO 19600: ISO 19600 provides guidance on compliance management systems and can be used as a framework for developing and implementing compliance programs.

8. World Health Organization (WHO):

- WHO Guidelines: WHO publishes guidelines on various aspects of healthcare, including clinical practices, patient safety, and research ethics.

9. Healthcare Compliance Association (HCCA):

- HCCA Resource Library: HCCA offers a variety of resources, including articles, webinars, and toolkits, covering different compliance topics and best practices.

10. Health Insurance Portability and Accountability Act (HIPAA) Resources:

    - HIPAA Privacy Rule: Official guidance and resources provided by the U.S. Department of Health and Human Services (HHS) Office for Civil Rights (OCR) on compliance with HIPAA privacy regulations.

    - HIPAA Security Rule: OCR resources and guidance on compliance with HIPAA security regulations, including safeguards for electronic protected health information (ePHI).

11. Office of Inspector General (OIG) Compliance Resources:

    - OIG Compliance Program Guidance for Hospitals: Detailed guidance from the OIG on compliance program requirements for hospitals, including recommended elements and best practices.

    - OIG Compliance Resources: Various resources provided by the OIG, including compliance program guidance for other healthcare settings, advisory opinions, and compliance toolkits.

12. Centers for Medicare and Medicaid Services (CMS) Resources:

    - Medicare Learning Network (MLN): MLN offers educational resources, webinars, and training materials on Medicare billing, coding, and reimbursement compliance.

    - Medicaid.gov: The official website for Medicaid provides resources and guidance on compliance with Medicaid program requirements and regulations.

13. Drug Enforcement Administration (DEA) Resources:

    - DEA Diversion Control Division: The DEA offers resources, guidelines, and regulations related to controlled substances, drug diversion prevention, and compliance obligations for healthcare providers.

14. Federal Trade Commission (FTC) Resources:

    - FTC Health Breach Notification Rule: Guidance and resources on compliance with the Health Breach Notification Rule, which requires certain businesses to notify individuals and authorities in the event of a data breach involving personal health records.

15. State Regulatory Agencies:

    - State-specific Health Departments and Boards: Many states have their own regulatory agencies and departments that provide guidelines, regulations, and resources related to healthcare compliance. Check your state's official website for specific resources.

16. Professional Associations and Organizations:

- American Health Lawyers Association (AHLA): AHLA offers resources, webinars, and publications on various healthcare compliance topics, including fraud and abuse, privacy, and compliance program development.

- American Medical Association (AMA): AMA provides resources, guidance, and toolkits on medical ethics, billing and coding compliance, and other relevant topics for healthcare professionals.